Exploring Your God-Capacity as the Path to Your Destination

—————— THE ——————
HIGHER CHOICES COMPASS

LAURA ZUBER

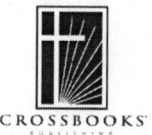

CROSSBOOKS
PUBLISHING

CrossBooks™
A Division of LifeWay
1663 Liberty Drive
Bloomington, IN 47403
www.crossbooks.com
Phone: 1-866-879-0502

First published by CrossBooks: 06/26/2012

ISBN: 978-1-4627-1712-5 (sc)
ISBN: 978-1-4627-1711-8 (e)
ISBN: 9781-4627-1710-1 (hc)

Library of Congress Control Number: 2012907631

Printed in the United States of America

This book is printed on acid-free paper.

ACKNOWLEDGEMENTS

I would like to express my sincere thanks to my dear friends for their contributions:

To Wendy DiNicola for capturing the essence of this book in her cover illustration; www.WendyDiNicola.com;

To Cindy Olszewski for being my mentor, and encouraging me to read all manner of theological and mind-stretching books;

To Barb Angell for teaching me to pray out loud, and what a friend really is;

To Linda Williams for encouraging my music, recognizing gifts I didn't know I had, and being my running partner (26.2!);

To Lisa Moreland for tireless interest in what I might have to say, encouragement, and being my photographer.

INTRODUCTION

*God has never created anyone just like you or me, and
the process of unfolding our Christ-nature is distinctive
with everyone. There is no clear blueprint known ahead
of time to follow, no precast mold into which to pour
ourselves. Each of us is an adventure of God's Spirit.*
– Tilden H. Edwards Jr.

The quote you just read by Tilden Edwards is practically the only introduction this book needs. Read it again, slowly, and ponder four key concepts, four reasons to discover the power of Higher Choices.

1. "God has never created anyone just like you or me," – God created each person to fulfill a unique purpose in this world, in his or her lifetime. Your originality is a gift.

2. "...the process of unfolding our Christ-like nature..." – Unfolding is a beautiful word to describe the transformation from our human nature to our ultimate destination to be like Christ. Like a blossom that opens and expands to become a beautiful flower, your transformation will expose the true beauty within as false perceptions are laid aside.

3. "There is no clear blue print known ahead of time…" – We live in a world governed both by God's will and free choice. You must find your own way, one day at a time, but God promises those who seek will find.

4. "Each of us is an adventure of God's Spirit." – The most exciting, fulfilling, surprising life adventure belongs to those who boldly embrace their calling, fueled by God's Spirit to operate at full God-capacity. Your function is your joy.

God-capacity is admittedly an odd term. Yet if you allow your imagination to create a mental image of this concept, you will see how magnificently it models Christian living. God-capacity is a person's actual and potential ability to be everything God created her to be. God endows His children with the capacity to perform all of life's functions, and to experience all of life's pleasures. God created us all to fulfill a purpose. It is my experience and firm belief that we realize abundant life to the degree our daily 'operations' are consistent with our unique individual designs, joyously embracing who we are, and performing our special work.

The word 'capacity' more aptly describes what we are in Christ than the word 'potential.' Capacity exists in everyone right now, whereas potential is yet to be. Looking at the definitions[1] and synonyms of each make this apparent:

- Capacity – the ability to receive or contain; actual or potential ability to perform, yield or withstand. Synonyms are: ability, competency, adequacy, genius, gift, inclination, power, qualification, skill, strength, talent.

- Potential – possibility for achievement; capable of being or becoming; latent excellence or ability that may or may

1: All word definitions from http://dictionary.com

not be developed. Synonyms are: conceivable, dormant, inherent, possible, probable, undeveloped, unrealized.

I studied engineering in college. When I think about capacity, I envision a large steel pipe designed to carry a specific volumetric flow. It may not always be full, but the capacity is inherent and always available. It is strong, able to withstand the pressure of its environment. The pipe does not produce the fluid - it is merely a conduit. Realizing your God-capacity means you know your designed function, defined by your gifts, talents, and genius, and you allow God to flow through you, benefiting your territory. It is His strength, power, and ability at work.

The Higher Choices Compass is a guide for discovering your God-capacity, and opening yourself to possibilities. **Higher Choices** are **your wisest, best choices for you to be consistent with God's will for you and the life God's enabling you to co-create.** Your God-capacity is within you now. However, you must do two things to effectuate it: know your purpose, and choose to live it. The exciting thing to grasp is the idea that your purposeful life is not really like that pipe at all, a precast form with limited utility. No, as Christians, you and I possess the freedom and authority to create our own lives. As we choose God's way, embracing our unique function in this time and place, we position ourselves to co-create the most fulfilling life imaginable.

I see two main benefits of living God's purpose for your life: **self-actualization**, and **fulfilling relationships**. Self-actualization, defined by Maslow in his book <u>Toward a Psychology of Being</u>[1] is "the desire for self-fulfillment, namely the tendency for him [the individual] to become actualized in what he is potentially. This tendency might be phrased as the desire to become more and more what one is, to become everything that one is capable of becoming." Making Higher Choices takes us beyond self-actualization toward Christ-likeness, to become actualized in everything God created us to be. The key word in Maslow's definition is 'desire.' Self-actualizing people want to fulfill their God-capacity, their destiny, and that intention drives their daily choices.

Fulfilling relationships are what life is about. We are relational people, thus the many rewards of relationships are the motivators for most of our choices about who to be and what to do. Although we all have family and friendship connections that exist regardless of our awareness or pursuit of a life mission, there is an extraordinary phenomenon I call **Connection and Direction** you experience as you live on purpose and stay open to God's leading:

Connection – the bonds through which meaningful relationships thrive.

Direction – the heading that aligns your life journey to your destination.

The quality of any relationship depends upon the strength of the connection. The essence of your connection with God will determine the condition of your connections to family, friends, co-workers, clients, etc. As you discover your purpose and pursue it as your life course, you will strengthen your connection with God and the special people He has placed on your path. Then, these connections affect the next directions your life takes. Affiliations become avenues to new choices. An easy example is whom you choose to marry. As life partners, you agree to collaborate on important decisions about family matters, including what city to live in, what neighborhood within that city, where to worship, how you spent your money, to only name a few, all setting your life direction. Through the influence of others, you encounter opened doors to new opportunities, a mixture of life-long dreams and wonderful unforeseen possibilities you would not have conceived of on your own. Although connections have a great affect on your direction, it is your choices that determine where you are headed and what that journey will be like. Many factors influence your choices. Choices about the environment you place yourself within and the lifestyle you choose determine your direction. So do your time management decisions, and the use of your talents. Your openness to new ideas and promptings of the Holy Spirit are factors, as well as your courage to be authentic and follow your heart's desires.

Making Higher Choices leads you to be everything you were created to be, and expands the quality of your relationships.

How to use this guide

The Higher Choices Compass coaches you through an adventure of self-discovery and spiritual transformation to nurture your God-capacity. There are two uses for a compass: 1) determine direction, and 2) measure distance. On your adventurous life journey with God, you will need to do both. As with any journey, the questions you ask, both in preparation and at strategic points along the way, are:

- Where am I heading?

- How far do I have to go?

- How do I get there?

Orientation is your ability to ascertain your true position relative to true north. The Higher Choices Compass presents twelve **Orientations**; principles and practices for discovering your path and sticking to it. The 12 Orientations include the eight bearing points on the front cover, plus four supporting topics, the former indicated below in italics:

1. *True North* – Reference point for life's journey; God the Father, Son, and Holy Spirit

2. Higher Choices – Paradox of free choice and God's supremacy

3. Ask, Seek, Knock – Process for discerning God's will

4. Prayer and Meditation – Connection to God

5. *Destination* – Gifts, Mission, and Vision

6. *Course* – Plan to reach your destination

7. *Priority* – Investment of time, money, and human resources

8. *Fitness* – Physical, mental, emotional, and spiritual wholeness

9. *Progress* – Personal development and spiritual formation

10. *Navigation* – Directional observation and course management

11. *Authenticity* – Natural creative genius and influence

12. Relationships – Fulfillment and motivation

Each orientation introduces four **Turning Points**, ideas or principles to consider adopting that lead to Higher Choices. Each has the following components:

- *Objective* – focused goal or desired result; an intermediate destination point along the course

- *Position* – location or place; attitude or opinion; belief or value

- *Exploration* – aids to analyzing how your position compares to the objective, whether or not adopting the stated objective fits your destination, and specific steps to take to test or put into practice.

Working through the Exploration questions allows you to coach yourself. I recommend keeping a journal to record all of the insights and ideas you encounter as you embark on this adventure of learning more about what you want, what God wants, and how to know the peace that passes understanding when these align. There are 48 Turning Points. Consider reading and working through one each week. May God bless you as you embark on your new adventure.

TRUE NORTH

Thy Word is a lamp unto my feet and a light unto my path.
— Psalm 119:105 (KJV)

Orientation 1: Trust and rely upon
God as your True North.

A compass is a valuable tool for reaching a destination, because it provides a reliable and consistent reference point - True North. You must trust the compass reference point for it to be an effective tool for your navigation. For the Higher Choices Compass, there is no difference between magnetic north and true north. In fact, God is like a magnet, always drawing His children close.

The Higher Choices Compass promotes biblical principles, supplemented with practical, real world methods and examples. Use it to determine your current life position relative to your God-given destination. Consider the principles it teaches in light of the direction your present life philosophy is taking you. Then adjust your course as you are called. You may be asking yourself if you have a defined personal life philosophy. Looking at the definition of philosophy, "the rational investigation of the truths and principles of being, knowing, or conduct," one can see that what she thinks, believes, and does reveals her philosophy – her position.

True North on the Higher Choices Compass is God. Through scripture, He reveals Himself to us as three persons: the Father, Son, and Holy Spirit. The churches of Christian tradition record and recite various faith statements to communicate their fundamental belief in

1

the Holy Trinity, or the Triune God. Recently, I have become familiar with the term "Godhead." I prefer to use this term, because it conjures a mental image of unity of purpose, and equality in power.

The Bible is the story of God creating and relating to humankind. By studying The Bible, we learn about God. We discover God's plan for His people. We come to know God both through our intellect and through experience, with the latter being the more enduring and tangible. It takes one's entire lifetime to fully know God and mature in relationship with Him. There is no way that I can fully describe God in this guide! What I can do, however, is describe ways you and I relate to God for the specific purpose of being available for Him to work in and through us for our own good, and the good of others. In so doing, we align our lives with God, and participate in co-creating with Him the abundant life He offers.

Our ultimate destination is God Himself, to be in His presence, and in His kingdom. I think, however, that God created this big round beautiful earth for us to enjoy and explore with Him. As we learn and grow into the persons God would have us become, we undoubtedly will traverse in many directions. The value of the Higher Choices Compass is to help us know our bearing relative to True North, so we can determine how to stay on course, reach the immediate objectives before us, and progress toward our earthly destination. Allowing God to determine the direction for your life requires faith in God as your source of truth. This Orientation highlights the special ways each member of the Holy Trinity operates as True North.

The four Turning Points you will consider in this Orientation are:

1. Orienting to True North – Make God your reference point in all decisions; your standard for daily living.

2. God the Father – Rely on the heavenly Father as your source for every good thing; to provide, protect, nurture, and defend.

3. God the Son – Become a disciple of Jesus Christ, and let Him show you the way.

4. God the Spirit – Listen to and obey the promptings of the Holy Spirit, the source of all wisdom and truth.

Make Higher Choices by orienting to True North.

Turning Point 1 – Orienting to True North

All we like sheep have gone astray;
we have turned every one to his own way.
– Isaiah 53:6 (KJV)

Objective: Make God your reference point in all decisions, your standard for daily living.

Position: Orientation is synonymous with direction, bearing, and goal. The Objective statement in each Turning Point is a goal for you to consider for fostering Higher Choices. Adopting each objective as a principle or practice helps you set the direction for your life. You choose to head in a certain direction, and then take steps to get there. To orient is also synonymous with adaptation, meaning to impart knowledge of a new thing or situation. For example, I attended freshman orientation with my daughters to learn about university expectations, and get a glimpse of what campus life would be like. Therefore, as we orient our lives to God, we choose to do two things: adopt and follow God's ways, and work to increase in wisdom and knowledge of His kingdom.

A compass helps you chart a course to your destination. With True North as your constant reference point, you can confidently determine your heading, ensured that you are moving in the right direction. Before you can reach any objective, you have to know your position, where you are relative to True North. The Position section in each Turning Point prompts an analysis of your attitude and opinion of the Objective, so you can consider embracing it as your own value or belief.

The prevalence of Global Positioning Systems (GPSs) makes finding our way to a new destination so easy that we readily forget the manual steps required. The satellite receives a signal telling it your current position. The maps associated with your general location are stored in the device's memory. With two pieces of data, where you are (Point A) and where you want to go (Point B), it uses the map to plot the direction you should take. There is usually more than one way to get there, so the GPS calculations default to the preferences you established. Once the GPS presents a route, you are ready to put the car in gear, and begin your adventure. When we are in unfamiliar territory, it is amazing how easy it is to choose the wrong road, or take a wrong turn. If your experience with this device has been anything like mine, then you have heard the friendly female voice kindly inform you of your mistake by saying, "Please drive the highlighted route," and "Recalculating," Oh, how I wanted to throw "her" out the window! However, it is not the GPS's fault when I fail to follow the directions. I am the one responsible for transposing the map and "her" instructions to the real-world terrain I wish to navigate.

The "Lost" TV series was a source of great entertainment for two of my children and me. A group of plane crash survivors, now stranded on a tropical island, encounters much controversy, challenge, confusion, even death in their quest to return home. They do not know where they are. There are other groups of people on the island involved in strange activity, so they are unsure whom to trust! Even after a few manage to make it back home, those individual's life choices cause them to remain "lost."

Throughout the Bible, we see how lost God's people become when they turn to anything or anyone else as their source of true direction. The Israelites wondered in the desert for 40 years before they reached the Promised Land, because they failed to follow the

Lord's instructions. Lot chose the better land in which to dwell when Abraham offered him first choice, but living among the heathen in Sodom and Gomorrah proved to be too great a temptation for his family to overcome to remain righteous. Samson, wanting to prove his love for Delilah, got lost by sharing the secret to his strength, and quickly suffered his ruin.

Thankfully, scripture tells of those who stayed on track and fulfilled their purpose because they remained aligned with God. Daniel is a great example, along with Joshua, Joseph, and many more. You will increase your capacity to love and serve God when you take time to observe and become fully aware of your position (Point A), and determine what thoughts or actions are required to align with your destination (Point B). The first step is agreeing that True North is your reference point, the standard that guides your decisions.

Exploration: Reflect upon your current position, bearing, and reference point.

1. To what places are your current mindset and habits leading you? Are you closer to where you think God wants you to be?

2. Can you identify any past decisions you made that caused you to be lost for a while?

3. What small directional changes and adjustments are you sensing you should take at this time?

> *Blessed are all who fear the Lord,*
> *who walk in his ways.*
> *— Psalm 128:1* [2]

2: Unless otherwise stated, all scripture references come from the New International Version (NIV), Red Letter Edition, Zondervan, Publishing House, 1985.

Turning Point 2 – God the Father

The young lions do lack, and suffer hunger: but they
that seek the LORD shall not want any good thing.
– Psalm 34:10

Objective: Rely on the heavenly Father as your source of every good thing; to provide, protect, nurture, and defend.

Position: Certainly not everyone has had a loving earthly father who has been a good role model to emulate. If you have had a negative parental experience, try to set that aside. Instead, consider what you imagine the perfect father or mother to be like. What characteristics would he or she have?

A great parent is wise; able to guide, protect, and provide; strong, reliable, patient, fun to be with; and comes running whenever you call. A parent's main job is to nurture a child until he or she is full-grown, equipped with sound mind, body, and spirit to live in this world. Parents want to pass on lessons life experiences have taught them and guard their children from harm. They also want their children to know the true sources of joy and happiness.

What does it mean to have a heavenly Father? How do you come to trust God the Father to show you the way and provide all you need? Throughout the Bible, we see that God views human begins as His children. The following Bible stories remind me of God the Father's good parental qualities (certainly not an exhaustive list):

- Wise teacher – the book of Proverbs is a collection of wisdom teachings to promote daily godly living. The primary lesson is on the benefits of obtaining wisdom herself.

- Protector – one of the most fantastic stories of God's protection is that of Daniel in the lion's den. Many children love this favorite story, even us big kids. The Passover in Egypt and Jesus as the Passover Lamb are promises of God's protection.

- Provider – the story of Joseph shows how God set Joseph in a position of power to save the Israelites long before they experienced a seven-year famine. God ensures that His people have everything they need.

- Adventurer – David and Goliath and Jonah and the big fish come to mind, as does the story of Jesus walking on water and casting Legion into a heard of pigs!

I am fortunate to have great parents that not only provided well for my siblings and I, but also made our childhoods fun and interesting. If we needed help with Math, we went to Daddy; English was Mother's specialty. Our parents taught us to care for ourselves, solve problems, and be independent. We enjoyed camping vacations, and fun family traditions. No Oklahoma winter was complete without eating freshly fallen snow like Cream of Wheat with milk, sugar, and butter, or roasting marsh mellows over the fireplace flames (I can't believe Mother let us do that in the house!). They made sure we received a good education, and supported us in school activities. We had fun learning about family history through entertaining stories. And thankfully, Mother and Daddy helped build for us a sure faith foundation by sharing their personal beliefs, and taking us to church were we could learn about and experience faith for ourselves.

Accepting God as Father means that we accept our role as children. Jesus said, *"Let the little children come to me, and do not hinder them, for the kingdom of heaven belongs to such as these"* (Matthew 19:14). Jesus teaches that we must be like little children in order to enter the kingdom of heaven (Matthew 18:3-4). What does that mean? What characteristics do children typically display that we can emulate? Dependence, a sense of wonder, energy, trust, unconditional love, and humility (sometimes) are a few. I am discovering that as I choose to become more dependent upon our heavenly Father, I am free from the burden of having to do "it" all by myself. I feel secure in God's provision and guidance, receive God's love, and learn to love God in return as he blesses me with every good thing.

In <u>Anointed, Redeemed, Transformed, A Study of David</u>[51], Kay Arthur, Beth Moore, and Prescilla Shirer do a wonderful job of guiding their audience in discovering God's overwhelmingly loving and compassionate nature by telling the story of David and Bathsheba. Kay shows the many wonderful qualities of the heavenly Father that enable David to approach God after committing many sins. We read in 2 Samuel Chapter 11 about David's transgressions of adultery, conspiracy, cover up, and murder. Once Nathan confronts David to show him the magnitude of his sin, David falls before the Lord in true repentance. Psalm 51 records his heart-felt prayer of confession and rededication. David remembers that God repeatedly demonstrates His steadfast love, loving kindness, compassion, tender mercy, and faultless judgment. The story of David's realization of how much God has blessed him and his family (1 Samuel Chapter 6), along with God's response to David's sin (2 Samuel Chapter 12), reveal to us how truly loving God is toward His children. The book of 2 Samuel tells of God's promise to David prior to David's "fall," and how God is faithful to fulfill that promise. David has just returned the Arc of the Covenant to Jerusalem. He looks around, appreciating the blessings of a comfortable home, and desires to honor God by building a beautiful home for "God's presence." God speaks to David through the prophet Nathan, clarifying that David is not to build a house for God, but that God will build a house, a nation, for him, through his son. Nathan declares:

> *"'The Lord declares to you that the Lord himself will establish a house for you: When your days are over and you rest with your fathers, I will raise up your offspring to succeed you, who will come from your own body, and I will establish his kingdom. He is the one who will build a house for my Name, and I will establish the throne of his kingdom forever"*
> *(2 Samuel 7: 11-13).*

David's indiscretion with Bathsheba occurs much later. The son she bears dies, but they have another son. He is to be named Solomon, the king who ultimately builds the Jerusalem temple. God is faithful to His promise to David and his household, despite the sin, because David is fully repentant, returning in worshipful obedience to the Lord. Speaking again through the prophet Nathan, God explains to David how much he is loved, and how much the Lord desires to bless the *"man after his own heart."*

> *"I anointed you king over Israel, and I delivered you from the hand of Saul. I gave your Master's house to you and your Master's wives into your arms. I gave you the house of Israel and Judah. And if that had been too little, I would have given you even more"*
> *(2 Samuel 12:7-8).*

What truly abundant love, mercy, and blessing! God loves blessing you more than the most loving parent does. But, you must discover this for yourself. As you make Higher Choices, you increase in obedience, which in turn positions you to receive more of God's blessings and experience God's presence on a consistent, daily basis.

Exploration: Experience God the Father by becoming like a child; care free, joyful, expectant, and trusting.

1. To what or whom do you currently turn for protection and provision?

2. What advice or direction do you need right now, that you can offer to God for solution?

3. What child-like mannerism can you adopt in your approach to God?

> Make a joyful noise unto the LORD, all ye lands.
> Serve the LORD with gladness:
> come before his presence with singing.
> Know ye that the LORD he is God: it is he
> that hath made us, and not we ourselves; we are
> his people, and the sheep of his pasture.
> Enter into his gates with thanksgiving, and into his courts
> with praise: be thankful unto him, and bless his name.
> For the LORD is good; his mercy is everlasting;
> and his truth endureth to all generations.
> – Psalm 100:1-5 (KJV)

Turning Point 3 – God the Son

Jesus said to them, "Very truly, I tell you,
before Abraham was, I Am."
– John 8:58 (NRS)

Objective: Become a disciple of Jesus Christ, and let Him show you the way.

Position: As mentioned early, most church congregations recite an affirmation of faith to communicate their fundamental beliefs. They acknowledge Jesus to be God's only son, who came to reconcile us to the Father through the forgiveness of sins. He was crucified, dead, buried, and arose from the dead that we might have everlasting life. He is Redeemer, Savior, and Friend. The Bible tells us in the first chapter of the book of John "*In the beginning [before all time] was the Word (Christ), and the Word was God himself... .And the Word (Christ) became flesh (human, incarnate) and tabernacled (fixed his tent of flesh, lived awhile) among us; and we [actually] saw his glory (His honor, His majesty), such glory as an only begotten son receives from his father, full of grace (favor, loving-kindness) and truth*" (John 1,14 AMP). Jesus shows us "The Way" by literally bringing God's truth to life.

You may wonder how Christ can effectively show you the way in everyday things. Jesus said, "*Come, follow me*" (Matthew 4:19). What does that really mean, and how do you do that in today's world? Would you go on a journey of any great distance with someone you just met? No! You and I are only willing to follow a trusted friend with a proven track record. Since the Godhead embodies all that is God, in the context of Higher Choices, following Jesus means following His example. Jesus' followers are called disciples. It was a youth pastor at St. Andrew's United Methodist Church in Plano, Texas, that gave the best description of a disciple I have ever heard. He said that the Greek word for disciple does not just mean follower, but is more accurately translated as "apprentice," someone learning what the master knows in order to become like the master. I thought of Arthur and Merlin; Luke Skywalker and Yoda! Disciples of Jesus Christ do not just follow; they are intentional in continuous transformation into His likeness.

Jesus is the most trusted friend you could choose to follow. You can trust Jesus because he was fully human, yet fully divine. He has been through whatever you have been through, so He understands. I can guess what you are thinking, particularly if you are a woman: "He has not been through everything I have experienced." No, Jesus did not experience every possible human situation or circumstance while He walked this earth, but certainly He experienced the full range of emotions all humans share. Jesus is worthy for you to align yourself with Him, because scripture tells us He only does what the Father tells Him (John 5:19). Jesus said, if you know me, you know the father. He is the Word come to life to open our eyes that we might truly see God.

The first time I really started to understand Jesus was through a Bible study by Maxie D. Dunnam, entitled <u>Jesus' Claims - Our Promises</u>[16]. It explains the "I Am" sayings of Jesus; I Am the Bread of Life, I Am the Good Shepherd, I Am the Door, I Am the True Vine, You Say That I Am a King, I Am the Resurrection and the Life, and I Am the Alpha and Omega. Much of Jesus' teaching is in word pictures and stories that provide clear examples of what God is really like. We can learn a lot about who Jesus is by examining these "I Am" pictures.

13

As the Good Shepherd, Jesus promises to care for our every need; to come find us when we wonder off; to ensure that we will know His voice. Like the Father, Jesus watches over, protects and nurtures His sheep. As our shepherd, He "lays down his life" for us, and promises to search for and find every lost sheep. The image of the Door, or Gate, is particularly helpful, because a gate both opens and closes. It keeps some things in, and other things out. Perhaps this is the most literal image of Jesus being 'The Way." We must go through Him to reach the greener pasture and still waters. It is by following His example that we are freed from attitudes and behaviors that pen us in. As we step through the gate into His kingdom, the gate closes behind us, allowing us to shut out any unpleasant past experiences and former ways. He also closes gates before us to seal off directions we should not take, keeping us from wrong choices that may lead to a treacherous wilderness. As the Bread of Life, Jesus urges us not to be concerned about whether or not our physical bodies are cared for, but to look to Him for setting the priorities of the day. Jesus will sustain, empower, and equip us to live a peaceful and joyful life in this world as we obey Him and keep His commandments. By saying, I Am the Resurrection and the Life, Jesus tells the disciples He has triumphed over death for all who believe. It is not enough to teach of His resurrection as a one-time event, but to extend the hope that we too are resurrected in Him when we allow Him to live in and through us.

My next major revelation of Jesus came through watching the movie The Gospel of John[15]. Seeing a real man portray Jesus, and hear him say repeatedly "*I tell you the truth...*," brought the scripture to life. Seeing the joyful, loving expressions on His face when interacting with people, and noticing the way He carried Himself made me simply, finally, fall in love with Jesus. Now this is only a movie, but the powerful images communicated Jesus' characteristics more personally. The easiest way to follow someone is to learn by example. A teacher or mentor can talk to you at length, and you will learn a great deal. However, when that same teacher demonstrates the principle, you grasp the concept much more quickly, and at a deeper level. You have a mental image to recall any time you need it. When you go further and put the principle into practice yourself, you build it into your character and life style. You will learn more about that in the Ask, Seek, Knock Orientation.

Choosing to become Christ-like is the way to abundant life. Paul wrote in his second letter to the Corinthians, "*Therefore, if anyone is in Christ, he is a new creation; old things have passed away; behold, all things have become new*" (2 Corinthians 5:17). You are making Higher Choices when you choose to think, speak, and act as Jesus did.

Exploration: Read the Gospel of John. Let Jesus speak to you.

1. As you read the Bible, what characteristics of Jesus are you noticing for the first time, or understanding more deeply?

2. How can you think and behave in a similar way? Be specific.

3. In your everyday encounters ask, "What would Jesus do?" (Trite, but effective.)

The Spirit of the Lord [is] upon Me, because He has anointed Me [the Anointed One, the Messiah] to preach good news (the Gospel) to the poor; He has sent Me to announce release to the captives and recovery of sigh to the blind.
– Luke 4:18 (AMP)

TURNING POINT 4 – GOD THE SPIRIT

*When the Friend comes, the Spirit of Truth, he will take
you by the hand and guide you into all the truth there is.*
– John 16:13 Message

Objective: Listen to and obey the promptings of the Holy Spirit, the source of all wisdom and truth.

Position: What do you believe spirit is? What is spirituality, or what does it mean to be spiritual? Lately it seems more people are seeking spirituality. There is a yearning to connect with a higher power as the source of meaning, guidance, and energy. The challenge is that the myriad of books, teachers, and self-proclaimed experts promoting "spirituality" make it difficult to know exactly what that means. As a member of the Godhead, the Holy Spirit is eternal, playing a significant role in both the Old and New Testament narratives. The Bible tells us the Holy Spirit is God's presence in the lives of New Testament believers, to empower, teach and guide Christ's disciples in fulfilling their purposes. The book of Acts tells the story of the early Christian church's growth. We read of the day of Pentecost and many following instances of the Holy Spirit's dynamic working in the lives of individuals and groups to grow the church, and further God's kingdom. The following passages illustrate this point:

- Acts 2: 20 (Message) – *This is what the prophet Joel announced would happen:*

"In the Last Days," God says,
"I will pour out my Spirit
on every kind of people:
Your sons will prophesy,
also your daughters;
Your young men will see visions,
your old men dream dreams.
When the time comes,
I'll pour out my Spirit
On those who serve me, men and women both,
and they'll prophesy.
I'll set wonders in the sky above
and signs on the earth below,
Blood and fire and billowing smoke,
the sun turning black and the moon blood-red,
Before the Day of the Lord arrives,
the Day tremendous and marvelous;
And whoever calls out for help
to me, God, will be saved."

- Act 8:26-30 – *Now an angel of the Lord said to Philip, "Go south to the road—the desert road—that goes down from Jerusalem to Gaza." So he started out, and on his way he met an Ethiopian[a] eunuch, an important official in charge of all the treasury of the Kandake (which means "queen of the Ethiopians"). This man had gone to Jerusalem to worship, and on his way home was sitting in his chariot reading the Book of Isaiah the prophet. The Spirit told Philip, "Go to that chariot and stay near it." Then Philip ran up to the chariot and heard the man reading Isaiah the prophet. "Do you understand what you are reading?" Philip asked.*

As a human being, you have a spirit, that unseen part of you; your "heart," if you like. In the Sermon on the Mount, Jesus says, *"Blessed are the poor in spirit, for theirs is the kingdom of heaven"* (Matthew 5:3). When you diminish your own spirit and yield to God's Spirit, you operate in love, creativity, energy, and knowledge – all of the Fruits of the Spirit. Connecting with the Holy Spirit as your life source allows you to experience much of the kingdom of heaven here on earth.

Beth Moore says the Holy Spirit shows us what is not obvious, and puts up road signs to keep us on track[30]. How appropriate that image is for understanding the Spirit's role as Truth North on our compass! The Holy Spirit is our ever-present guide, sharing words of wisdom, reminding us of God's truths we already know, and nudging us to consider new possibilities that may not be obvious. John 16:13 calls the Holy Spirit the "Friend." You know how great it is to have a trusted friend to whom you can turn in times need. When you are confused, want help with decision-making, or just need a little comfort and reassurance, God is present through the Holy Spirit.

To orient to True North via God's Holy Spirit, you must be receptive, actively listening, as if tuned into your favorite radio station. There are many biblical references to the *"still small voice."* Elijah found God in the *"sound of a gentle whisper,"* not the loud wind, earthquake, or fire (I Kings 19:11-13). Yet rest assured, for the one who truly seeks, God makes Himself known through the Spirit. I love the line from a song by Out of the Grey that says:

> "He is not silent
> He is not whispering
> We are not quiet
> We are not listening"

Your job in properly orienting yourself is to do what you can to tune in. That means adjusting your receptivity. Distraction is a major obstacle to staying in tune with the Spirit within and around you. You can reduce this "static" by using the tools in this Compass on a consistent basis. You know what to do! Regularly read the Bible. Spend time in prayer and meditation. Ask for discernment. God, through the Holy Spirit will guide, fulfill, and sustain you.

Exploration: Be receptive to the Holy Spirit. Notice and eliminate distraction.

1. What promptings or suggestions are you receiving from the Holy Spirit? How are you taking those ideas and putting them into action?

2. What practice or discipline can you adopt now to boost your receptivity?

3. Notice what appears throughout the day to distract and divert you from. What do you hear the Holy Spirit suggest is an alternative to that?

But when the Holy Spirit controls our lives, he will produce this kind of fruit in us: love, joy, peace, patience, kindness, goodness, faithfulness, gentleness and self-control.
– Galatians 5:22-23 (TLB)

HIGHER CHOICES

What happens when we live God's way? He brings
gifts into our lives, much the same way that
fruit appears in an orchard – things like affection
for others, exuberance about life, serenity.
– Galatians 5:22 (Message)

Orientation 2: Realize true abundance as you
co-create with God, one choice at a time.

Making Higher Choices demonstrates your agreement to be the person God intended, and takes you above the level you are currently living to a new plane. "Higher" is an appropriate adjective to describe the choices we make consistent with God's will. The dictionary gives several definitions for the word higher: exceeding the common degree or measure, strong; exalted in rank, station, eminence etc.; of exalted character or quality. Isaiah 55:8 tells us, *"'For my thoughts are not your thoughts, neither are your ways my ways,' declares the LORD"* *(NKJ)*. Most of us equate higher with better – higher quality, higher standards. Stevie Wonder had a hit song entitled, Higher Ground[62], where he sings about continuing to pursue a purer, more spiritual life. In one of the most inspirational books I have read, <u>The Power of Intention</u>[17], Dr. Wayne Dyer describes enlightened beings who live with intention as being higher energy people. Low energy thoughts and emotions are anger, fear, depression, etc., but higher energy thoughts (and resulting behavior) are love, kindness, compassion, and the like. Wayne says that Jesus was the highest energy person who walked the face of the earth. I would agree with that!

The choices you make are yours and yours alone. Only you can decide what you want and need, and what is higher for you in any given circumstance. God's will for you is not the same as God's will for anyone else's at the level of daily living. The Bible clearly tells us God's general will for all of humankind. It is the same for every individual. *"Jesus replied, 'Love the Lord, your God, with all your heart and with all your soul and with all your mind.' This is the first and greatest commandment. And the second is like it: 'Love your neighbor as yourself.' All the Law and Prophets hang on these two commandments"* (Matthew 22:37-40). These simple instructions tell me the right attitude to have - how to conduct myself. However, they are not illuminating enough to provide specific, practical guidance for knowing and fulfilling my God-capacity, my purpose. Higher Choices is a process for seeking and realizing God's will for you on a moment-by-moment, decision-by-decision basis. Higher Choices enable you to live out your personal calling, and become your best self. The seemingly routine, daily choices you make are the building blocks of your life. What are you building?

The four Turning Points you will consider in this Orientation are:

1. Pay Attention - Understand and appreciate the value of daily choices, and who or what influences them. Consider aligning your choices with God's will.

2. God's Will - Know and desire God's will for your life by seeking to know and desire God.

3. Free Choice - Recognize the wonderful power and possibility you receive through God's gift of free choice

4. Life is an Adventure - Look forward to the abundant life Christ offers anticipating excitement, embracing surprises and uncertainties.

Become a co-creator with God, and allow Him to take your life to a new level. The exciting, and frankly, uplifting realization you have is that allowing God to direct your life is to have the Creator of the Universe as your partner! You are not alone, and you do not have to do anything by yourself. You and I have the most powerful, wealthiest, influential, kind, and loving partner showing us the way and supplying our every need. We only need to ask, and be willing to follow.

Turning Point 1 – Pay Attention

*No trumpets sound when the important decisions of
our life are made. Destiny is made known silently.*
– Agnes De Mille

Objective: Understand and appreciate the value of daily choices, and who or what influences them. Consider aligning your choices with God's will.

Position: The majority of what you become and do in life is of your own choosing, a result of all of your decisions, large and small. Events and circumstance occur in our lives that are beyond our control. However, you and I do have control over our responses to what life presents to us. Brian Tracy teaches his students to say, "I am responsible." Yes, that can be a tough pill to swallow! It is easier to blame others for our less than desirable circumstances. When you can embrace this truth, you realize that better choices create a better life. Whether it is deciding your day's priority tasks and appointments, choosing your response to another's actions, or deciding what to eat for breakfast, taking a few seconds to consider if your choices are consistent with the person God calls you to be is the most practical way I know to truly live your faith and experience abundance.

Making Higher Choices consists of three steps. First, pay attention - be aware that you are *always* in a position to choose. Choices are almost as prevalent and continuous as the air you breathe, taking the form of a decision you need to make, a response to a person or event, or accepting an opportunity presented to you. Increasing your self-awareness and paying attention to your surroundings will heighten your sensitivity to choice opportunities. For example, before you chose what to watch on television last night, you first chose to spend time watching television. When you decided to cook a special family breakfast last weekend, you chose to be creative, be of service, and show your loved ones they are a priority in your life. We make bad choices too, of course. Those hurt feelings you experience are because you chose to take offense at what somebody said or did. Second, once you realize you have a choice to make, pause for just a moment to search your heart for Higher Choices. Your life experience and knowledge guide you well, but Higher Choices come from asking God for guidance. Checking in, so to speak, to test your motivations and to imagine the results of your choices before you make them, gives you clarity. Deep down you know the right choice for you. Third, make the choice! Your power is in action. Peace comes from making end roads along what you know to be the wisest, best course for you.

Exploration: Pay attention to all your daily choices, both large and small.

1.   Notice the number and quality of your choices, and the results they produce. How full is your schedule? Are you getting enough rest? What is the quality of your food and drink choices? What are you thinking about? How do you interact with friends, family, and people you meet?

2.   Observe how others influence your decision-making. For whom are you making the choice?

3.   Listen to your inner voice. Where is she guiding you?

> But blessed are those who trust in the Lord and
> have made the Lord their hope and confidence.
> – Jeremiah 17:7-8

TURNING POINT 2 – GOD'S WILL

*God does not reveal God's will to the curious but to
the obedient. Faith is obedience without reservation.*
– Disciple I Bible Study

Objective: Know and desire God's will for your life by seeking to know and desire God.

Position: Higher Choices are those that are consistent with God's will to the degree you discern that at any point in time. Many events you observe in life, whether they are world events that shake nations, or personal events that require you to alter your life course a bit, seem to occur at random and make little sense. You may question if God has a specific will and plan for anyone's life.

I was leading a women's small group at our church in Pittsburgh when the September 11, 2001 terrorist attack against the United States occurred. In the weeks that followed, the group's discussion focused on the pursuit of justice. The main question posed was "Should the United States participate in the war (we are still fighting), or should we follow Jesus' command to turn the other cheek, i.e., seek a peaceful resolution over retaliation? What is God's will in this situation?" Questions like these illustrate how the great uncertainties and complexities of life in this world can cause us to doubt God is in charge, or that there is a right or wrong way to do anything.

My mentor at that church loaned me a book entitled <u>The Will of God</u>[58], by Leslie D. Weatherhead. Weatherhead's logical and clear explanations brought great peace and comfort to me. It enabled me to reconcile the conflict in my mind between believing that God's will prevails, while knowing that simultaneously, people everywhere are free to think, do, and say what they want. Weatherhead says that confusion arises when we say "the will of God" without distinguishing between three types of God's will -- three ways it is realized.

- God's Intentional Will - God's ideal plan for man (humankind)

- God's Circumstantial Will - God's plan within certain circumstances wrought by man's evil

- God's Ultimate Will - God's final realization of His purpose; nothing of value lost; God is sovereign

You may want to read this book. Nevertheless, the simple, straightforward approach for you to know God's will is to come to know God. This is the message of the quote from Disciple I Bible Study[60], and the overarching message of this book. Think of some of the people closest to you. You often know their will, because you know them intimately. You can probably say without a doubt how they would feel about a certain situation or decision. I have searched many stores to buy a golf shirt with a front pocket for my dad, because I know that is the only kind he really likes. Understanding God's will, I believe, works much the same way. Go beyond just being curious about God as some far off deity and establish a relationship. Knowing God positions you to know God's will for your life. You will begin to see, as I do, that you would not want it any other way.

As we seek to make Higher Choices, the difficulty in discerning God's will is not just our lack of understanding about who God is, but also who we are. How can you make a choice that will take you to a higher level of happiness if you do not know what makes you happy? How can you make a choice that will let you realize your full capacity if you do not know the gifts and talents your posses? This is the adventure! As you apply the tools in the Higher Choices Compass, you begin the journey of discovering who you are, who God is, and what the two of you can be and do together.

The quote above communicates another key principle – the importance of obedience. Not only is obedience required to both be entrusted with knowing God's will and receiving all you need to carry it out, but it is through the act of obedience that you and I increase our trust in Him. The more you know God, the more you love God. Then you more earnestly seek His presence and influence in your daily decision-making. Henry Blackaby and Claude V. King produced a fantastic study entitled, <u>Experiencing God, Knowing and Doing the Will of God</u>[5]. They present what they call Seven Realities of Experiencing God. Number 7 is "You come to know God by experience as you obey Him and He accomplishes His work through you." It is in an earlier section, however, that they describe the link between love and obedience. They point to John 14:21, where Jesus says, *"Whoever has my commands and obeys them, he is the one who loves me. He who loves me will be loved by my Father, and I too will love him and show myself to him."* Jesus demonstrated His perfect love of the Father by obeying Him. He could do that because he knew the Father's nature to be love. I appreciate how Blackaby and King put it: "Never in your life will God ever express His will toward you except that it is an expression of His perfect love. He can't! He can never give you second best." So it is that as you obey God, you learn, appreciate, and love His ways. Staying aligned to True North allow you to sustain a beautiful, life-long relationship where you continually grow closer to God as you make progressively Higher Choices.

Exploration: Review what you know about God, and what you would like to know.

1. The Bible is the story of God relating to His people. It reveals God's character to us. Select a few Psalms, read them, and identify the characteristics of God you identify.

2. Meditate upon Romans 8:28 and Jeremiah 29:11. Do you know the purpose to which you are called?

3. What do you want to know about God?

4. Are you comfortable with the paradox that God is in control, yet you know you have free choice? How do you think obedience enters the "equation?"

Don't copy the behavior and customs of this world, but let God transform you into a new person by changing the way you think. Then you will know what God wants you to do, and you will know how good and pleasing and perfect his will really is.
– Romans 12:2 NLT

TURNING POINT 3 – FREE CHOICE

Freedom is not merely the opportunity to do as one pleases; neither is it merely the opportunity to choose between set alternatives. Freedom is, first of all, the chance to formulate the available choices, to argue over them – and then, the opportunity to choose.
– C. Wright Mills

Objective: Recognize the wonderful power and possibility you receive through God's gift of free choice.

Position: Accepting total responsibility for our lives is difficult. We can accept some of the bad things we experience when we believe they are beyond our control. The ancient Greeks and Romans believed the mythical gods controlled every aspect of their lives, both good and bad. They resigned themselves to the belief that another determined their destiny. If you take a poll today, you will get a variety of responses regarding what people believe about God and fate. Do your choices matter? Is your destiny within your control?

Our heavenly Father has blessed the human race with a most precious gift — choice. The magnitude of the freedom and power to choose is difficult to accept, for along with this gift comes the responsibility to live with the results and consequences. Freedom of choice expresses God's perfect love. God wants a relationship with us. He desires that we choose to love, listen, obey, and rely upon Him. Don't you feel most loved by the people in your life when they *choose* to spend time with you, or do things for you? You know they care for you when they take time to get to know you, and express concern for your wellbeing. It is God's desire that you choose to love and worship Him. God takes the initiative, but the choice to respond is yours.

The challenge for believers in exercising free choice is feeling secure that you are aligning yourself with God's will. My husband and I endured a lengthy decision process to choose his new job a few years ago. From the beginning, we both sought and prayed for wisdom and discernment about God's will for our future. A new job choice ultimately affects the lives of our children, our extended family, friends, and both of us. It would be easy if my husband only received one job offer. Then it would seem as if God's will had prevailed. Fortunately, he had at least three sound opportunities from which to choose. Which one was God's will? Any of them could be! The choice was ours.

Apart from conscious, intentional acts of wrong-doing or neglect, whether the outcomes of your choices are deemed good or bad is simply your judgment about the outcome. Wayne Dyer has much to say about this in his fine book, You'll See It When You Believe It[18]. He writes, "You relate to everything and everyone on this planet through the mechanism of thought. It is not what is in the world that determines the quality of your life, it is how you choose to process your world in your thoughts." You will learn more about thought in the Fitness Orientation. Consider here that free choice is available to us, because the process of connecting with God and listening for God's voice is most important. Did you get that? The *process* of seeking, studying, and listening to God demonstrates your love and obedience. When you trust God to be faithful and show the way, you are able to exercise your will and choose with confidence. Within the boundaries of God's law, not acting out of selfish motives, but actively seeking godly council, God's will can indeed be a wide road upon which you can exercise much free will. You have the power and grace to co-create abundant life through Higher Choices.

Exploration: Examine what you believe about free choice, fate, destiny, and God.

1. What are your ideas about fate, destiny, and God's will?

2. People who really love you will support you in your choices. Do you think a loving God does the same?

3. Choice is freedom. Do you think your ability to choose is limited in some way?

4. How do you feel about the statement "You are the sum of all of your choices to date?"

> May we think of freedom, not as the right to do as we
> please, but as the opportunity to do what is right.
> – Peter Marshall

TURNING POINT 4 – LIFE IS AN ADVENTURE

It is expectation make a blessing dear; heaven
were not heaven if we knew what it were.
– Suckling

Objective: Look forward to the abundant life Christ offers anticipating excitement, and embracing surprises and uncertainties.

Position: When I think of adventure, I imagine a journey to some new, exciting place that offers the elements of beauty, surprise, wonder, and fun. An adventure should be something thrilling. To say, "life is a journey," sounds boring, as if it takes a lot of time and effort!

I have found that my life has a good element of adventure the more I trust God with my choices, and seek God's ideas. Some of my best experiences have involved people, places, and things I would never have thought of. God knows us better than we know ourselves, thus He knows what delights us. Laurie Beth Jones provides an excellent example of this in <u>The Path</u>[30] video lessons. She tells the story of a four-year old boy who throws a fit in the ice cream store, where he and his mother have come to select a cake for his birthday. He is mad that she said "no" to his request for the ice cream cake he saw on the bottom shelf. He resists her as she tries to pick him up, too distraught to let her finish her sentence. "No, Jerod. This one," she says as she lifts him kicking and screaming to a higher shelf where he can see the cake she selected. "Dinosaurs!" he exclaims, with great delight, as his pain and suffering vanish. Often we are like that boy, willing to settle for the first thing we see, not realizing that God has something much better planned for us; something He knows will delight us completely.

A friend and I were recently talking about the progress of new a ministry project, and we both commented about how God continues to amaze us both, all of the time! When we are open to the possibilities, amazing things happen. God gave us our sense of adventure, and I think God relishes opportunities to have us join in the many expeditions and explorations available.

There are at least three key elements to adventure: *anticipation, trust,* and *uncertainty.* I love the roller coaster at MGM Studios theme park in Florida, called "Rockin' Roller Coaster." The ride is exciting because it is mostly dark, the room only lit by neon highway signs and the reflective lines on the "road." It takes you through many twists and turns, hills and valleys, with wind-in-your-face speed, while Aerosmith rocks in your ear. You *anticipate* fun and excitement, and that is what you get. Why isn't the ride scary? There is *trust.* The riders having the most fun completely trust that the designer and builder did their jobs well. The ride is safe and enjoyable because it has been perfectly orchestrated, programmed when to turn, when to slow down, and when to shed just enough light. The first time on the ride is the most thrilling, due to *uncertainty,* the element of surprise. Riding many times is fun, but the adventure tapers once you know what is coming.

I don't think people allow God to guide their life too much, because they don't give God enough credit for being the Great Adventurer who can create more fun and excitement in their life than they could ever imagine. Consider removing the limitations you place on your life, because you have placed those limits on God. You will experience many little adventures, get "off the ride," and say "Wow! That was cool! Let's go again."

Exploration: Add excitement and wonder to each day, trusting that God will let you in on some little adventures.

1. Is there a normal activity you could do differently this week to add excitement, like cook a new recipe, take an excursion, or read a really different book?

2. Creating adventure requires you to release control and step out of your comfort zone. What are you not willing to try, but would like to? What is holding you back?

3. Where can you begin to trust God more with great anticipation?

It is very difficult to generalise.
Everyone's adventure is original.
– Bernard Pivot

ASK, SEEK, KNOCK

More often than not, they (words from God) will
be utterly practical instruction about seemingly
trivial matters, for God wants us to live out our
spirituality in the ordinary events of our days.
— Richard J. Foster, Celebration of Discipline

Orientation 3: If you truly want to
know God's will, simply A.S.K.

There are no quick and easy formulas for discerning God's will. It is more important to be in a relationship with God than to set about trying to accomplish some lofty goal, as if it were just another item to check off your already too long task list. What really matters is the motivation behind your desire to know God's purpose for your life, and the process of Connection and Direction your seeking will take you through. Given that, there are sound principles you can trust to guide your thoughts and actions if you truly want to realize your God-capacity. It occurred to me that perhaps the process for discerning one's purpose is described by Jesus as Ask, Seek, and Knock (A.S.K.). We read in Matthew 7:7 what Jesus said in the Sermon on the Mount, *"Ask and it will be given to you; seek and you will find; knock and the door will be opened to you."* Believing that the Bible is our instruction book for living in today's world, how do we apply these steps to enjoy the blessings of kingdom living?

Learning to exercise your faith to rely upon God as your True North, and trusting the guidance you receive to live according to His will, is similar to other learning processes. The steps are:

- Establish communication – through prayer and meditation, ask God to show you the way.

- Increase in knowledge – study God's Word, and learn all you can

- Be receptive to new ideas – pay attention to insights and godly wisdom from a variety of sources

- Make small changes – act upon simple ideas

- Test new outcomes – observe and evaluate the results of your choices and resulting actions in light of your objective question

- Make improvements – adjust the process to your unique needs and circumstances

- Stick with what works – practice and perfect your truth

The four Turning Points you will consider in this orientation are:

1. Ask - Learn God's will for you by asking a variety of questions relating to all areas of life.

2. Seek - Willingly dig beneath the surface, see beyond the first glance, and test ideas that reveal God's truth.

3. Knock - Discover God's personal truth for you, persevering in practice until it becomes part of you.

4. Abide - Experience the joy of living a new truth by remaining connect to the One who makes all things possible.

This is a logical sequence of events. Each step is more earnest and expansive than the previous. The words *ask, seek,* and *knock* are so familiar it seems the process should be intuitive, and that all people would recognize this simple process's inherent power. However, conscious and consistent thought and prayer are essential aids to each step. You are asking God to help you become the best "you" possible. You are asking God to reveal more of Himself and His will for you. There are, therefore, some attitudes to consider in approaching God in this way. God bids us come before His throne of grace and enter into His kingdom. I identify two key attitudes God teaches in scripture: come with expectation, and come in obedience.

Expectation

"How great is the love the Father has lavished on us, that we should be called children of God! And that is what we are" (I John 3:1)! We are God's beloved children. Recall that this position is described in the True North Turning Point, God the Father. Every child not only expects a loving parent to meet their needs, but to anticipate and exceed their desires as well. John tells us in the scripture quoted above that God's love for us is lavish. There is a wonderful song by Casting Crowns that echoes this, entitled Your Love Is Extravagant[11]. The chorus has the following text:

> Your love, it is extravagant
> Your friendship, it is intimate
> Spread wide in the arms of Christ is a love that covers sin
> No greater love have I ever known
> You considered me your friend and captured my heart again

Because you and I were created by God, He indeed does know our needs, and meets them before we ask, often exceeding them in peculiar and spectacular ways. After Jesus tells the disciples to *ask, seek,* and *knock,* the very next words are, "*Which of you, if his son asks for bread, will give him as stone? Or if he asks for a fish, will give him a snake? If you, then, though you are evil, know how to give good gifts to your children, how much more will your Father in heaven give good gifts to those who ask Him*" (Matthew 7:9-11)! We get what we expect out of life. Positive expectations lead to positive experiences. The reverse is also true, i.e., positive experiences breed positive expectations. You and I can count on God, because "*The Lord is gracious and compassionate, slow to anger and rich in love. The Lord is good to all; he has compassion on all he has made*" (Psalm 145:8-9).

Obedience

"*Dear friends, if our hearts do not condemn us, we have confidence before God, and receive from him anything we ask, because we obey his commands and do what pleases him.*" (1 John 3:21-22) Jesus told the disciples that those who love God show it by obeying His commandments (John 14:15). There are two ways we can be disobedient: 1) failing to do things we know we ought, and 2) doing things we know we should not. God requires obedience as a prerequisite for bestowing blessing upon blessing. The fifth chapter of Deuteronomy details how Moses received the law from God, the Ten Commandments. After God showed the Israelite people "his glory and majesty," they promised to uphold their side of the covenant. In verse 28, Moses tells them, "*The Lord heard you when you spoke to me and the Lord said to me, 'I have heard what this people said to you. Everything they said was good. Oh, that their hearts would be inclined to hear me and keep all my commandments always, so that it might go well with them and their children forever...*" (Deut 6:28-29) Further, Psalm 25:10 says, "*All the ways of the Lord are loving and faithful to those who keep the demands of his covenant.*"

Attempting to know and do God's will can be disquieting, for we are never quite sure we understand Him and His ways. We have doubts that cripple our initiative. However, Jesus promises that those who seek will find. Learn how the A.S.K. process, a very simplified description of the complex interplay between knowledge and faith in the one we trust (True North), will lead you to Higher Choices. Trust that the more you A.S.K., the more you find God helping you create the life that's good and best for you and those you love, influence, and serve. You may have read or heard this scripture many times before, but it is a timeless truth:

"We are assured and know that [God being a partner in their labor] all things work together and are [fitting into a plan] for good to and for those who love God and are called according to [His] design and purpose" (Romans 8:28, AMP).

Turning Point 1 – Ask

*Being religious means asking passionately
the question of the meaning of our existence
and being willing to receive answers,
even if the answers hurt.*
— Paul Tillich

*Ask and it will be given to you; seek and you will
find; knock and the door will be opened to you.*
— Matthew 6:17

Objective: Learn God's will for you by asking a variety of questions relating to all areas of life.

Position: "Oh God, please tell me what to do!" How many times have we thought or uttered those words in desperation, seeking some insight from above to alleviate a crippling fear or uncertainty? Often people wait until they have become desperate, or have exhausted themselves and their personal resources, before they turn to God. What would happen, however, if you realized that God is ready and able to respond to what you may consider your most mundane, routine question? What would you step out and accomplish if you had at your disposal the greatest source of wisdom, a loving guide with your best interest at heart? How many more choices would you let God influence?

God's purpose for your life is rarely revealed unsolicited. Remember the context here is increasing our capacity for God by actively choosing to know His will. If you do not know, then ask. Ask God about your job, relationships, family goals, and personal desires. Every time you encounter opportunities to make meaningful life choices, whether it comes from desire, vision, knowledge, opportunity, challenge, or loss, is a chance to ask God to shed a little more light upon your path.

All of your knowledge comes to you in one of two ways: reading or hearing something presented to you, or seeking information to answer a question. All of your decisions begin with a question within your mind. For example, you may routinely ask yourself questions similar to the following, albeit unconsciously:

- What time shall I wake tomorrow?

- I wonder if I can afford to buy that right now?

- What should I eat for lunch?

- Should I accept that invitation to the party this weekend?

- Where do we want to go for vacation this summer?

To whom are those questions directed, and from whence does the answer come? That may depend upon the urgency and importance of your need, and the time available. Of course, you and I rely largely on our personal storehouse of knowledge and experience. We are not aware of the constant inner dialogue of question-answer, question-answer, because our habits and instincts are quick on the draw! Nevertheless, the fact is that we ask ourselves a question to evoke a decision. Taking time to be aware of these steps, and then considering what the Holy Spirit may suggest is the beginning of the A.S.K process. You can most likely answer the sample questions above without any advice or assistance. Decisions that involve other people will require you to consult with them, or you may seek some objective advice to help you make an important choice.

I propose that making a conscious effort to align your choices with True North requires you to heighten your awareness of decision-making opportunities, so you can actively seek God's input into the process. All too often we act out of habit, or unconsciously, perhaps with only short term implications in mind. That is not bad necessarily. In his very interesting book, Blink: The Power of Thinking Without Thinking[22], Malcolm Gladwell explains, "Our unconscious is a powerful force. But it's fallible. It's not the case that our internal computer always shines through, instantly decoding the "truth" of a situation. It can be thrown off, distracted, and disabled. Our instinctive reactions often have to compete with all kinds of other interests and emotions and sentiments. So, when should we trust our instincts, and when should we be wary of them? Answering that question is the second task of Blink. When our powers of rapid cognition go awry, they go awry for a very specific and consistent set of reasons, and those reasons can be identified and understood. It is possible to learn when to listen to that powerful onboard computer and when to be wary of it." You and I have many good habits, and the majority of daily decisions are not worth agonizing over. However, if you want to improve some aspect of your life, if you want to know and fulfill your purpose, then asking questions is the place to begin.

I John 5:14-15 says we can approach God with confidence because we know he hears us when *"we ask according to his will."* Wait a minute! Doesn't that sound like a "chicken or the egg" problem? How can I ask according to God's will if that is precisely what I am trying to figure out? To me, it simply means being open to receiving God's will, however it may be revealed. The point is to be conscious of how many opportunities arise each day to connect with God and obtain God's guidance. The more specific the question, the more specific the response will be. God is interested in every aspect of your life, and wants to be a part of it all. Asking is a catalyst for divine connection. Your resulting relationship with God will increase your ability to approach Him with confidence, and be receptive to what God's will for you may be.

Asking God to co-create your life takes two types of questions. One is asking questions for which you are looking to God as your decision-making partner. You have a choice to make. It may be large or small, but in your desire to be obedient and please the Father, you ask Him to give you an idea for the direction He wants you to take. The second is making a petition for some favor or blessing, some way that God will act in and among your circumstances to fulfill a need or desire. This request may be for yourself or a loved one.

Two of my favorite authors and inspiring people, Tony Robbins and Laurie Beth Jones, both instruct on "the power of the question." In her book, Jesus, Life Coach[29], Laurie tells us that Jesus used open-ended questions to provoke transformation in His people. She writes, "We can sit and read or hear a lecture all day long, but never really take in the material. When we are called upon to answer questions about the material, that means some 'registration' has gone on." She also says that open-ended questions convey respect, connection, and continuation. To promote what he calls CANI (Continuous And Never-ending Improvement), Tony Robbins says, "If you want better results, ask better questions." Tony explains the importance of the wording of your questions, because questions can presuppose an answer. For example, if I ask myself "What can I learn today?" I have set up in my mind the condition of being aware of and receptive to opportunities for learning something new.

I have defined A.S.K. as the process for making Higher Choices, and experiencing abundant life. You may wonder, like me, why we need to ask if God loves us and is waiting to supply our every need. Here are some of the reasons I suspect God has ordained it this way:

- Relationship – Asking initiates the connection and conversation. Then, as you and God continue in dialogue, you get some ideas and work with God to discover your truth. Spending time with God builds your relationship.

- Submission – Asking recognizes God as the authority in your life. Eliciting His input into your decision-making process shows God respect by asking His opinion.

- Self-discovery – Asking requires you to articulate what you want. If you do not know, then asking is the way to discover your deep desires.

- Humility – Asking means you admit you do not know something, and that you need help.

- Child-like Inquisitiveness – Asking displays a sense of curiosity and adventure, and opens the door to exciting ideas you would otherwise miss.

- Vulnerability – Asking allows God to care for us. You relinquish control and allow God to direct your choices.

Just as there are many reasons to ask God to reveal His will and influence our lives through His favor, there are a few reasons why this can be difficult. Reluctance is born out of doubt, fear, and a sense of unworthiness. Doubt prevents us from looking beyond our own limitations to a God who has none. You know you cannot do it, thus find it hard to believe that God can. Perhaps fearing the disappointment you will experience in finding out that God's plan is different from yours keeps you from asking. Think how much easier life would be if you could step out in a faith, so sure and confident that nothing would be too hard for you in partnership with God. Faith is indeed liberating. Television, books, and movies recount story after story of those "lucky" folks who experience miracles, because they first had the faith to believe God enough to ask that their prayer be answered. If they receive the answer they were looking for, then why not you, and why not me? Perhaps you do not think you deserve it. You are not sure if your desires fit within God's plan. It is safer, emotionally, not to set yourself up for disappointment. Your suspicion that prayers are seldom really answered may indeed be confirmed, and that would be too much to bear. I love the way Beth Moore has such high expectations for God moving in her life. There is not anything she does not think God can do! I read her retelling of the story of Joshua's battle against the Amorites, in her book Believing God Day by Day: Growing Your Faith All Year Long[34]. The Israelites were outnumbered five to one. Joshua had the audacity to ask God for not one, but two huge miracles. The Israelites where fighting hard at Joshua's command, but the day was wearing on. Darkness soon would come – a sign of sure defeat in a foreign land against this foe. So, backed by his bold faith in the Lord, Joshua asked God to stop the sun until the battle could be won. Do you believe that? Stopping the sun from moving across the sky, as it has every day for eons, like a ship stuck in autopilot, is the boldest request I have ever heard of. But, guess what? Yes, God did it. He did it for Joshua, for the Israelites, and for God's own glory and renown.

In Matthew 21: 21, Jesus says, *"I tell you the truth, if you have faith and do not doubt, not only can you do what was done to the fig tree, but also you can say to this mountain, 'Go throw yourself into the sea,' and it will be done. If you believe, you will receive whatever you ask for in prayer."* Yet in the garden at Gethsemane, Jesus *" fell with his face to the ground and prayed, 'My Father, if it is possible, may this cup be taken from me. Yet not as I will, but as you will.'"*

You can feel confident asking God to show you Higher Choices with just a few simple steps. First, study scripture to understand God's commands and desires for all of His people, and allow that knowledge to formulate petitions and requests consistent with the Word. God told Joshua that he would defend him and defeat his enemies. It was in that context, i.e., his knowledge of God's promises, that Joshua made his request to have the sun stop. Second, surrender to a loving God, knowing that He always works toward our best interest. Accept that in the greater plan, small battles may be lost in order to pave the way for larger victories down the road. Third, know and pursue your God-given purpose, your God-capacity. It serves as a framework to keep you moving in the right direction, like rigid, steel train tracks. The range of uncertainty regarding God's will for our lives is reduced, enabling more focused and specific questions.

Exploration: Pay attention to the questions you ask yourself while making choices.

1. Specific questions lead to specific answers. Ask for detailed guidance relating to one immediate decision in each area of your life, such as work, family, leisure, community.

   a. Example: How much money from this new client should I give to honor God's provision to me, and to what organization?

   b. Example: How can I promote and encourage a more Christ-like attitude in my children?

2. Write 3 to 5 questions you could ask yourself each day to set up positive, expectant thoughts and actions that lead to Higher Choices. For example:

   a. What can I learn today?

b. How can I fit exercise into my schedule today?

c. How can experience fun, peace, and joy?

d. Where are you at work around me, Lord?

*This is the confidence we have in approaching God: that
if we ask anything according to his will, he hears us.*
– I John 5:14-15

TURNING POINT 2 – SEEK

Readiness is the opening God needs.
– Unknown

We cannot seek or attain health, wealth, learning,
justice or kindness in general. Action is always
specific, concrete, individualized, unique.
– Benjamin Jowett

Objective: Willingly dig beneath the surface, see beyond the first glance, and test ideas that reveal God's truth.

Position: We learn to walk before we run. I watched my children learn to walk by first grasping the coffee table or the leg of a chair to help them stand, then carefully taking small steps around it, still holding on. When they felt confident and brave, they let go of their support to venture out into the open space on their own. All three of them learned at different times, with varied senses of urgency. The process, however, was the same: take one step at a time, hold on for support as you practice, and then let go.

Seeking is taking the initial insights and ideas that come in response to your Asking, and putting them into practice. The old cliché "you'll never know unless you try" holds a lot of truth. With regard to making Higher Choices, sometimes the answer to questions such as "Why?" and "Is this God's will" are "Why not?" and "Perhaps." There is work to be done to discover the answer. When I first started

48

pursuing my certification in music ministry, it was not clear to me if that was part of my purpose. Seeking to know more, I learned that the program was four years of two-week summer school sessions. It was not expensive, nor terribly inconvenient. I asked myself, "Could I go for the first year and explore the potential of music ministry as a personal passion?" Sure! It only cost two week's time, a few hundred dollars, and my family's willingness to be slightly inconvenienced while I was away. That first year opened new, exciting doors, and answered major questions about God's purpose for me. Not complete answers mind you! I did not have a clue about what exactly I would be doing, where, or how. However, the blessings began immediately those first two weeks, and have continued beyond my imagination. What a shame it would be had I not been willing to try!

To seek means to find, discover, or look through carefully, experiment, delve, practice, uncover, and find by exploration. When you ask God to reveal His will, you receive ideas in the form of promptings from the Holy Spirit that you may try and test as potential partial answers to your questions. You may have a personal insight, or you may be inspired by a word from a friend. God uses many ways to communicate with us.

Two main precepts of seeking are: 1) God's will is revealed in manageable chunks, and 2) practice allows the idea to be tested and perfected. Seeking helps you discover:

- whether or not the idea is a good one (validation through a sense of peace and assurance from others),

- whether or not the principle or practice needs improvement (make modifications as necessary and test new outcomes), and

- what implications or outcomes to plan for.

God shows us the way one step at a time. Where you are heading, your Destination, is a broad vision that describes "what" your life will look like as a result of you living on purpose. "How" you get there is revealed in the ideas. Ideas are your objectives – a spark of insight that sheds light on your path. As you try some ideas and put them into practice, you gain clarity about the territory you are exploring. The outcomes produced by your actions indicate what works and what does not, allowing you to zero-in on the particular way you could implement the objective and how important it is to your life. Reaching one objective places you in a position to see more, perhaps better objectives as well. Just as you can see the mountaintop through the jungle's edge as the brush is cleared, seeking gives you the perspective and focus you need to identify your unique path.

Suppose that once we ask and are willing to wait and listen, God, through His Spirit, gives an answer. The answer is most likely not the whole picture, but will be enough to get us moving in the right direction. Answers, in the form of ideas, lead us to our next objective. Many of us have wonderful ideas of our own, yet few of us are truly experiencing the abundant life that living at our God-capacity brings. When I started working as a business coach, my partner and I established the foundation of our practice upon what we considered to be four progressive keys to success: Principles, Plans, Actions, Outcomes. For Higher Choices, the Bible gives us the *principles*. You will learn about *plans* in the Course Orientation. You must take *action* to make progress on your journey, and seeking is taking action. Jack Canfield, in <u>The Success Principles, How to Get from Where You Are to Where You Want to Be</u>[9], devotes eleven pages to communicating the necessity for taking action. He writes, "When you take action, you trigger all kinds of things that will inevitably carry you to success...Things that once seemed confusing begin to become clear. Things that once appeared difficult begin to be easier. You begin to attract others who will support and encourage you. All manner of good things begin to flow in your direction once you begin to take action."

Let me share a personal example of how I applied the A.S.K. process to determine how I could create a healthy exercise and eating guideline that allowed me to enjoy the foods I love. I formed the mental question "How can I take the best of many diet and exercise programs and tailor what is best for the body you gave me, Lord?" Having seen an advertisement in a Christian magazine for <u>The Maker's Diet</u>[47], I got the idea that I could research that reference without spending any money if I could find that book in the library. The book was available, so I checked it out, and began to read. This diet is too extreme for my chosen lifestyle, however, it did prod me to adopt the principle of reducing my consumption of pork and seafood – both described as the "garbage cans" of the earth and sea, respectively (not a particularly healthy or appetizing image). Another set of ideas came from a book entitled <u>Total Body Transformation</u>[28], by Steve Ilg. This very intense program combines challenging weight training, cardio, and yoga exercise routines with a spiritual approach to nutrition. I started practicing yoga, and learned how to engage my mind and emotions with both my nutrition and exercise practices. I can tell you that, although I love vegetables and eat a lot of them, I have no desire to be a vegetarian (tried that)! Thus, after just a few months, I have settled on a complete fitness framework that keeps me feeling and looking great. My current fitness vision statement (more on this in the Destination Orientation) says, "I enjoy a wide variety of foods and beverages in moderation." I credit God with giving me direction. He honored my request to honor Him with my body. I know that doing the work to which I am called and living well depend upon maintaining high energy and vitality.

Our society rewards effort. Effort spent seeking God is most certainly rewarded. *"Seek and you will find."* (Matthew 7:7) You will have to lift more than one rock and push aside some dirt, but you will find. Through the prophet Jeremiah, God promised the Israelite people that they would find Him if they sought with all their heart; *"'For I know the plans I have for you,' declares the LORD, 'plans to prosper you and not to harm you, plans to give you hope and a future. Then you will call on me and come and pray to me, and I will listen to you. You will seek me and find me when you seek me with all your heart"* (Jeremiah 29:11-13).

Seeking is stepping out in faith. Faith, according to Hebrews 11:1 (AMP), *"is the assurance (the confirmation, the title deed) of things [we] hope for, being proof of things [we] do not see and the conviction of their reality [faith perceiving as real fact what is not revealed to the senses]."* Exercising faith, you embrace an idea and expend effort confidently expecting a great outcome.

Living in the world means that you and I will always be subject to worldly ideas not consistent with God's will. I am not one to readily blame my mistakes and misfortune on the devil, but 1 Peter 5:8 warns us, *"Stay alert! Watch out for your great enemy, the devil. He prowls around like a roaring lion, looking for someone to devour"* (NLT). Thus, caution should be exercised in discerning godly ideas.

Let's revisit my earlier example of learning to walk. Understanding the need to move one foot in front of the, one at a time, is probably easy enough for a toddler to grasp. They have been watching their parents and others do it for months. Once they try this idea for themselves, daily practice fosters their discovery of all the intricate nuances. The child now must pay attention to balance, speed, arm movement, distance, floor surface, and the interaction of all these. Once she possesses basic walking skills, it is her persistent use of these skills that eventually produces her mastery. She can walk anywhere, anytime, without so much as a fleeting thought.

Applying the A.S.K. process to physical skills is indeed child's play compared to its application to living on purpose. Making Higher Choices is not a physical exercise. Higher Choices are decisions to align your thinking with True North, and take action consistent with God's will. Once you have asked questions and begun to receive

God's guidance, try a couple of ideas to test their validity in your life. Be willing to ponder and then act upon the promptings of the Holy Spirit to learn what direction God may want you to take. When you are consistently practicing the disciplines of prayer and meditation to stay aligned with True North, the Spirit will reveal what you need to know.

Exploration: Be receptive to ideas as potential answers to your questions and put them to the test.

1. Act upon seemingly small insights and intuitions to see where they lead.

2. Keep a journal of inspirational ideas and insights as they come to you.

3. Are there any ideas you sense God has revealed to you? How can you try one now?

4. What dirt and debris do you have to dig up and remove to put a great idea into practice?

> *One of The Secrets is that when you have an inspired thought, you have to trust it and act on it.*
> *– Jack Canfield*

Turning Point 3 – Knock

For nothing is hid, that shall not be made manifest; nor anything secret, that shall not be known and come to light.
– Luke 8:17 (ERV)

How often – even before we began – have we declared a task 'impossible?' And how often have we construed a picture of ourselves as being inadequate? ... A great deal depends upon the thought patterns we choose and on the persistence with which we affirm them.
– Piero Ferrucci

Objective: Discover God's personal truth for you, persevering in practice until it becomes part of you.

Position: Strange as it may sound, golfing and singing have both taught me a great deal about personal development and spiritual maturity. The biggest lesson may be just how long it can take to realize lasting improvement. Another is the power, confidence, and ease that infuse your performance of any task, once the principles and skills are ingrained in your body. Making progress requires a strong desire and commitment to hang tough when you encounter frustrations and setbacks. Sometimes once you gain progress, you encounter a hurdle that causes you to wonder why what was working last week is not working today!

The definition for knock is "to strike a blow; to make a pounding noise." This definition does not provide much insight other than to help us imagine that we probably will not get very far without using some energy and making a little noise! When I read the synonyms "persist" and "persevere," I knew that was God's message:

- persist (carry on or carry through, abide, repeat, endure), and

- persevere (keep at, work hard, be determined, go for it, hang tough).

Change is challenging! Jesus said, "Knock," to tell us we will have to be persistent and persevere.

Time spent practicing any skill allows you to take basic instruction and adjust the procedure so it is tailor-made for you. Voice and piano lessons taught me the significance of muscle memory. When you practice a physical skill, the repeated action trains your muscles, whether it is your vocal chords, diaphragm, or fingers, until they "remember" the appropriate sequence of movements and amount of pressure to apply. I have been singing long enough now that I can breathe deeply, using my diaphragm, and lift my soft pallet to sing with very little thought. Within the context of the A.S.K. process, knocking is the part where transformation takes place. It is the time, energy, and mental attention required to instill lasting change. I have been fascinated by the stories of the human mind's capability to unconsciously process information, enabling split-second decisions, as presented in Malcolm Gladwell's book, <u>Blink: The Power of Thinking Without Thinking</u>[22]. Knocking builds God's principles into our "default." As skills improve, performance increases in quality and ease, because muscles take over. Now, with your mind no longer completely occupied with mechanics, the door is opened and you are able to enjoy the process. It feels natural. It becomes part of you. It is your truth.

You have to persist in any endeavor when you see less progress than you like. You have to persevere when your head or heart knows what to do, but the actions you are taking just are not working for some reason. You have to persevere when your timing is not God's timing. Consider that the times when you are standing outside the door waiting and pounding are opportunities for your personal growth and transformation. God wants to build our character. Perhaps the times when we have to knock, God is getting us, and our circumstances, ready for the next step. Matthew 6:17 says, *"Knock and the door will be opened to you."* Persisting in learning God's truth will require some bold energy, and it may cause us to be a little noisy! What is it you are striking? Are you pounding on a door to new opportunity, or trying to knock out any undesirable habits you have allowed to develop through old thought patterns?

Adopting biblical principles and the specific ideas you glean from asking and seeking into your character and behavior requires endurance and patience. It takes energy, and it takes time. Time is an extremely important factor in successfully navigating a Turning Point that will lead to consistent Higher Choices. The Bible has much to say about the importance of waiting. Two noteworthy verses are Psalm 27:14, *"Wait for the Lord; be strong and take heart and wait for the Lord,"* and Psalm 130:5-6, *"I wait for the Lord, my soul waits, and in his word I put my hope. My soul waits for the Lord more than the watchmen wait for the morning, more than the watchmen wait for the morning."* Waiting allows time to build trust and faith in God. You will learn more about this in the Progress Orientation.

Knocking exercises faith. The greater the obstacle or challenge, the greater the faith required to overcome. The challenges we encounter in life grow, strengthen, and mature our faith – faith in God and ourselves. It is part of the human design that developing skill mastery comes from repeating an action until it is fully understood. When I was working as an independent software process consultant, I developed a training course for process improvement leaders. One lesson described the steps of the human process for adopting new methods, illustrated by a cartoon of sculling water bugs. Four frames lead you through their discovery that learning something new requires an open mind to receive instruction, acclimation to the environment where the new skill will be applied, but mostly practice, practice, practice in order to assimilate the skill to both mind and body.

Once you "get it," the new idea becomes a truth for you. Ingrained in your make-up, Higher Choices rarely require a concerted effort or conscious thought. You exude naturalness. This principle applies to both physical skills and matters of the soul – thoughts, emotions, and spirit.

Depending upon who you ask, it can take anywhere from 21 to 66 days to replace old habits with new ones. When you are able to stick with it and remain faithful, you will reap the rewards of owning a newfound truth for your life. Then, when the door does finally open, you will be ready! There are, and will be, difficult hurdles or obstacles through which you will have to "hang tough," but the overall sensibility is that of being in a divine flow. That feeling overrides the fear and doubt. John 16:13 says, *"When the Friend comes, the Spirit of Truth, he will take you by the hand and guide you into all the truth there is."* Trust that as you stay oriented to True North, the Holy Spirit will reveal the whole truth to you.

Exploration: Remain steadfast in persevering with new ideas and challenges.

1. Take one idea from the Seeking Exploration and take some action to practice it daily.

2. What obstacles can you remove by figuratively "striking a blow?"

3. Do you have an unrealized goal that simply did not receive enough time? Can you try again with more persistence?

I know the price of success: dedication, hard work, and an unremitting devotion to the things you want to see happen.
— Frank Lloyd Wright

Turning Point 4 – Abide

*I am the vine, ye are the branches: he that abideth
in me, and I in him, the same beareth much
fruit: for apart from me ye can do nothing.*
– John 15:5 (KJV)

Objective: Experience the joy of living a new truth by remaining connected to the One who makes all things possible.

Position: Surrendering to God and faithfully following His lead requires more strength and endurance than we possess. We must be willing to abide. Jesus explains the importance of staying connected to Him: *"I am the vine, ye are the branches: he that abideth in me, and I in him, the same beareth much fruit: for apart from me ye can do nothing" (John 15:5, KJV).* The image of the vine helps us see that we are to stay connected to Him to the degree that two become one. The vine supports and nourishes the branches so they can bear much good fruit. Abiding goes beyond fellowship to a state of intimacy with the Lord where you experience inner peace, strength, and motivation as you travel your path. This is what it means to say that Christ lives within you. You are a vessel, a conduit with high capacity.

As you Ask, Seek, and Knock, you discover some portion of God's will for your life. Then, the challenge is being faithful to this higher truth that the world perhaps does not recognize. Living transformed may be a challenge you face alone, without help or understanding from friends and family. You may even suffer persecution in some way. I was blessed last summer to read <u>The Cost of Discipleship</u>[6], by Dietrich Bonhoeffer. Bonhoeffer explains that only the faithful are obedient, and only the obedient are faithful. He writes, "If we are to believe, we must obey a concrete command. Without this preliminary step of obedience, our faith will only be pious humbug, and lead us to the grace which is not costly." Further, he says, "You can only learn what obedience is by obeying. It is no use asking questions; for it is only through obedience that you come to learn the truth." We start by asking the questions, but it is only by taking the ideas, the commands if you will, from God and persevering in obedience that we truly know the truth, and live it for the sake of Christ. The good news, however, is that God does not expect us to obey in our own power! In response to Jesus' saying that those who would follow him, deny themselves and take up their cross (Luke 9:23), Bonhoeffer offers, "To deny oneself is to be aware only of Christ and no more of self, to see only him who goes before and no more the road which is too hard for us. Once more, all that self-denial can say is: 'He leads the way, keep close to him.'"

Abide in Christ, and you gain His strength when you are weary; you feel his peace when you are nervous and anxious. Abiding increases your sensitivity to the Holy Spirit's suggestion for the next step to take when you think you have lost your way. Abiding gives you courage to continue the journey when you cannot see how to go on. Christ spoke to the woman at the well about living water (John 4:1-26). You and I must remain on the vine to be fully equipped and nourished. Unlike stagnant water in a well, living water is fresh, clear, energizing, satisfying, and always available. Jesus not only said, *"apart from me ye can do nothing,"* but also *"If you remain in me and my words remain in you, ask whatever you wish, and it will be given you. This is to my Father's glory, that you bear much fruit, showing yourselves to be my disciples" (John 15: 5,7,8 KJV).* The Amplified version of Paul's famous words in his letter to the Philippians says it well: *"I have strength for all things in Christ Who empowers me [I am ready for anything and equal to anything through Him Who infuses inner strength into me; I am self-sufficient in Christ's sufficiency"* (Phil 4:13).

The true disciple of Jesus Christ realizes that apart from Christ, she can do nothing. Traversing through the A.S.K. process with God brings a new awareness and appreciation for all God is doing in your life. You have a keener sense of awe and fear of the Lord. You bow before him in humble praise and thanksgiving. Seeing yourself as God's instrument of service, you acknowledge that your value and worth as a loving presence in this world is His gift to those whom you love, are connected with, and encounter in your daily rounds. You realize that you are magnificently capable in any endeavor, because Christ lives in you. You accept and receive daily the Holy Spirit's indwelling as a source of counsel, strength, power, and peace. Once you fully experience the fruit of this new truth in your life, you realize that the fruit only continues, as you stay connected to your source.

Creating lasting change in your life meets with opposition, both from within and without. There will be times when you are tempted to revert to old habits of thought, word, and deed. You will face challenges, either in your relationships with people who do not understand or embrace your new truth, or from the world in general. The next Orientation presents ideas for staying connected by spending consistent quality time in prayer and meditation. The Navigation Orientation presents tips for identifying and overcoming obstacles.

Exploration: Abide in the Lord as you travel along the path of truth.

1. What new truth and/or practice have you discovered that you need to stay with?

2. Who may be resisting your changed attitude and actions? How can you let abiding in Christ sustain you in "hanging tough?"

3. How is abiding revealing new blessings, and motivating you to continue progressing?

> *The personal life deeply lived always*
> *expands into truths beyond itself.*
> -- Anais Nin

Prayer & Meditation

Therefore let everyone who is godly pray to you
while you may be found.
– Psalm 32:6

Orientation 4 - Discover the many ways to
connect with God, your source of energy,
strength, peace, and understanding.

As with knowing God's will, prayer and meditation are large topics to present. There are many forms of prayer, and just as many interpretations of what constitutes meditation. I view these two disciplines as distinct, yet complimentary practices that overlap and intertwine.

The four Turning Points you will consider in this orientation are:

1. Conversation - Talk with "Abba, Father" in quiet, intimate conversation to release and receive.

2. Meditation - Meditate upon scripture to renew and re-energize.

3. Intercession - Praying for others is priority number one, not a last resort.

4. Worship - Exalt and worship the Lord in word and song.

63

Developing a consistent prayer life is essential to your faith. Spending time with God is foundational to every Turning Point within Higher Choices. The ways that you personally relate to God will evolve throughout life, so do not get discouraged by trying to accomplish too much too soon. Learn what others do, so you can take advantage of their experience. In time, you will figure out what works best for you.

A good prayer life is built upon discipline. You must set aside a specific time and have a specific place. Your prayers will be more effective if each you have a purpose and plan. Consider this as you read the Turning Points that follow.

TURNING POINT 1 – CONVERSATION

*Make prayer a habit, whether you recite the fixed prayers
of your tradition or the spontaneous words of your heart.
They are the lullaby of a restless soul.*
– Karyn D. Kedar

Objective: Talk with "Abba, Father" in quiet, intimate conversation
to release and receive.

Position: Conversation is the most direct and intimate form of
communication. Taking time to attentively listen and talk to another
person, one-on-one, is an act of love that feeds the relationship. You
exchange ideas, receive new information, and share your feelings.
Each person enjoys the company of the other. Good conversation is
responsive and engaging, not scripted.

What a privilege we have to be able to speak to God personally.
Beginning with The Exodus, Old Testament people relied upon the
priests to talk to God, hear God's Word, make their requests known,
and atone for their sins. Jesus' resurrection tore the veil of the Holy
of Holies, so all believers have access to God the Father through
Him (Matt 27:5). He shocked the Jewish people and religious leaders
when he addressed God as "Abba," which means "Daddy." Thanks
to Christ, you and I may have intimate, personal conversation with
the Lord of Hosts!

Conversational prayer with God should be informal and frequent.
By informal, I mean that as long as we approach the Father in

reverence, awe, and humility, we can share anything on our hearts and minds. The two-way exchange facilitates your ability to both *release* and *receive*. Release your sins, hurts, regrets, and burdens. Receive God's forgiveness, love, comfort, and guidance.

Although conversational prayer should be free-flowing, inspiring aids such as written prayers, room settings, and body postures all create an atmosphere conducive to prayer. If you don't know where to begin, perhaps you can try a prescribed prayer using specific words, or body postures similar to those described in Living in the Presence[19], by Tilden Edwards. I adapted one of his ideas to create my own conversational prayer, specifically to release and receive, by combining a "gesture" with a word phrase expressing my openness to God's presence, and readiness to receive what He might have to say to me. "Meaningful gesture can unite mind and body and present us whole to God," says Edwards. Here is an example:

Sit comfortably on the floor or in a straight-back chair. Rest your hands on the top of your thighs in a relaxed, natural posture. With your palms facing downward say, "Lord, I release to you …," stating the specific care you wish to release. Repeat these phrases as many times as you like in order to name each burden or concern the may be weighing you down. For example, I might say, "Lord, I release my apprehension about the class lecture I will give tomorrow." Or "Lord, I release my frustration over failing to hold my temper in last night's discussion with my daughter." Next, turn your palms facing upward, and in a similar fashion, let God know you are ready to receive a blessing to fill the new, open space created by the release. Continuing with the example above, I might say, "Lord, I receive your peace concerning tomorrow's class, knowing that you have guided my preparation, and you will be present with me, ensuring the message will touch someone in a special way." Likewise, the second release prayer may call for a receptive statement something like this: "Lord, I receive your forgiveness for expressing anger with unkind words. Be with me as I apologize to (person's name), and ask their forgiveness."

Release means to let go. Let go of your worries and concerns, for Jesus says our heavenly Father cares for us and knows our every need. Psalm 55:22 says, *"Cast your cares on the Lord and he will sustain you; he will never let the righteous fall."* Receiving can be as challenging as releasing. We must believe in order to receive. Faith in God's love for us allows us to accept God's forgiveness and every other good gift. Jesus tells us that everyone who asks receives.

There is a well-known prayer guide known as A.C.T.S. – Adoration, Confession, Thanksgiving, and Supplication. This acrostic presents the order of focus for what I am calling a conversational prayer.

- Adoration – Praise God and enjoy His presence. Think about the characteristics of God, all of the wonderful reasons He is to be revered and held high above all things. Speak the words of the Psalms. Be still and listen for the Lord to speak to you.

- Confession –We must first confess and repent in order to continue the conversation. Sin is a very personal matter. It may be difficult to know what to confess, or how to express what is on your heart. Ask the Lord to show you what displeases Him, and to reveal unknown sin. Repent and accept His forgiveness.

- Thanksgiving – We cannot thank God enough for the many blessings we receive. Counting blessings and acknowledging that all things come from the Father brightens your attitude. Examine all areas of your life and appreciate all you have been given. Thank Him for sustaining grace and salvation.

- Supplication – Go before God on behalf of others: family member, friends, co-workers, political leaders, teachers and schools, and the stranger you meet on the street. Be specific. It is a privilege to intercede on behalf of others. Ask God to fulfill your personal needs and desires also. Keep a list, so you can look back and see how your prayers were answered.

Learning the power of praying God's Word is new to me. The Bible is full of God's promises to His people. You and I can speak those promises to the Lord in prayer, thanking Him for granting such blessings, for who He is, and for being present in our lives. Two specific scriptures became my sustaining prayer last year, promises that both comforted and guided me as I recited them back to the Lord (AMP):

- II Chronicles 20:17 *"You shall not need to fight this battle, take your positions, stand still, and see the deliverance of the Lord [Who is] with you, O Judah and Jerusalem. Fear not nor be dismayed. tomorrow go out against them, for the Lord is with you."*

- Matthew 6:26-30 *"Look at the birds of the air; they neither sow nor reap nor gather into barns, and yet your heavenly Father keeps feeding them. Are you not worth much more than they?..."*

The Spirit guided me to these passages in my regular study time. Be receptive in your conversational prayer, so God can speak a special word to your heart.

Exploration: Whether you plan a time, or do it "on the fly," talk with God as if He were your best friend.

1. Set aside a specific time and a specific place for a few minutes of conversational prayer – daily if possible.

2. Select a Psalm or favorite scripture, and try rephrasing it into a personal prayer.

3. Pray the Release and Receive prayer when you feel stressed or worried.

4. Do you have any topics that are off limits for discussion in prayer, and if so, why?

5. What is your favorite part of spending time alone with God?

6. Have you been able to truly release your burdens and receive God's promises?

What happens in meditation is that we create the emotional and spiritual space which allows Christ to construct an inner sanctuary in the heart.
– Richard J. Foster

Turning Point 2 – Meditation

*I meditate on your precepts and consider your ways. I
delight in your decrees; I will not neglect your word.*
– Psalm 119: 15-16

Objective: Meditate upon scripture to renew and re-energize.

Position: Different faith traditions promote certain physical postures
and various ways to observe and manage your thoughts through
meditation. Richard Foster tells us that Christian meditation is
simply "the ability to hear God's voice and obey his word[19]," and
that the focus on obedience and faithfulness distinguish it from
other forms of meditation. A couple of years ago I read an article
that said that, because we use words to think, our thinking is limited
by our vocabulary. Such a profound statement this is, yet so true! As
I consider how I think, forming sentences with words and phrases
using my personal vocabulary, I am struck by the importance of
learning scripture. God's Word is God's vocabulary. Renewing our
minds and progressing toward having the mind of Christ (1Cor
2:16) will only be accomplished by knowing scripture.

Real understanding of God's Word comes when we are able to
internalize it, one or two verses at a time. For me personally, daily
devotionals are too frequent and short to facilitate deep understanding
and personal application of godly principles. Meditating upon just
one scripture for an entire week provides time to consider what God
is saying to me, and receive ideas for applying them to my life now.

The Bible study group I attended in Kuala Lumpur completed Rick Warren's study entitled <u>40 Days of Love</u>[56]. The way we approached this material called for little or no detailed daily study. We met weekly simply to view the DVD lesson together, and then discuss the topic in small groups. Rick presented five major love characteristics from 1 Corinthians 13: Love is Patient, Love is Kind, Love Speaks the Truth, Love is Forgiving, Love is not Selfish. Although Rick added many supporting scripture verses from other books in the Bible, all of these "acts of love" appear in verses 4-5. This was truly an exercise in meditation, since each participant was able to spend a whole week contemplating a specific portion of God's Word, and working out its implication in her world.

Spending a few days of actively living a single idea accomplishes many things:

- You begin to see through your interactions with others how the thought or command is manifest in reality; it takes on real form and shape in our relationships and circumstances

- You overcome obstacles and objections to new ideas by giving them time to prove promising

- You memorize the Word so it can be recalled as a source of comfort and strength in future times of trial and distress

- You develop habits that in the end, build your character.

In a nutshell, this is the A.S.K. process at work! You Ask God to reveal Himself and His will as you search the scriptures. You Seek ideas as you meditate upon that scripture for one week, and put it into practice in daily affairs. You Knock by persevering through obstacles to find the truth God has for you at this specific time.

Review how you currently spend your quiet time with God. Are you reading little snippets of scripture that easily go in one ear and out the other, or are you feasting on the rich bounty of God's message, savoring every bite?

Exploration: Infuse God's vocabulary into your mind through regular weekly meditation.

1. Have you ever pondered a verse for an extended period? Did it change your thoughts and actions?

2. What are you learning about God?

3. What are you learning about yourself?

4. What new words and principles have you adopted to guide your thoughts?

> I meditate on your precepts and consider your ways.
> I delight in your decrees; I will not neglect your word.
> -- Psalm 119: 15-16

TURNING POINT 3 – INTERCESSION

*We must begin to believe that God, in the mystery of
prayer, has entrusted us with a force that can move the
Heavenly world, and can bring its power down to earth.*
– Andrew Murray

Objective: Praying for others is priority number one, not a last resort.

Position: Coming before the Lord to pray on behalf of friends and family is a privilege. It is a powerful force for positive change. There are many times when you feel helpless to provide tangible help for someone in need. Perhaps someone is struggling with a challenge at work or school. Maybe your spouse suffers from a lingering illness. You may have a friend in mourning, and the words to comfort in time of grief escape you. Realize that you are far from helpless, because what you can do is pray, and that is noble work. Indeed, consider it your first response.

Richard Foster says, "The Bible pray-ers prayed as if their prayers could and would make an objective difference.[21]" Moses prayed that God would not destroy the Israelites after they built the golden idols, but rather God would spare them for His own glory. The apostle Paul repeatedly demonstrates the practice of intercessory prayer, not only praying for others (Eph 1:17, I Ti 2:1, Eph 3:17), but also asking that the church pray for him (Eph 6:18,19).

You cannot change another person, but you can ask the Father to move his or her heart toward change. Often in intercessory prayer, the person making the request is the one changed. For in asking God to act for others, we must believe that what we are asking is in line with God's will. Thus, we must ensure that our desires are not self-motivated. Is it your loved one's behavior that God should change, or your acceptance of that behavior as an act of love?

Some people have the spiritual gift of intercession. You may have the privilege to know someone with this gift. Sometimes their work is public, but often it is quiet and private. Several years ago, the senior pastor at our church in Pittsburgh started an intercessory prayer ministry. The feedback received from the spiritual gifts training they offered showed that many people had the gift of intercession. Coupling this with the understanding of the power and benefits of prayer, the senior pastor was inspired to develop a program to minister to both individuals and the church body as a whole. A key component of the ministry's success was the open publicity and education about the ministry to the church at large. The congregation saw prayer at work, positively affecting many lives. In my mind's eye I can see the green prayer cards made available to anyone anywhere in the church facilities: in holders on the back of each pew, stacked on the welcome table in the main hall, and next to the music slots in the choir room. Those submitting prayer requests simply filled out the card, and either placed it in the offering plate, gave it to an usher during worship, or most meaningfully, brought it to the basket at the altar railing during the singing of the prayer hymn, where one could kneel and pray as part of the worship service.

People serving on the intercessory prayer team pledged to come to the church at a specific time of their choosing to pray over a group of cards. Worshipers were told that their prayers would be lifted before God by one or more persons throughout the entire week. Additionally, the prayer team met as a group on a regular basis to support and encourage one another. They exchanged information and ideas to keep the ministry vital and effective. An annual tradition of arranging stacks of all the cards prayed over for the last year, and celebrating the importance and effectiveness of prayer in the life of that congregation was a powerful symbol of God's work in and around us, and a testimony to the faithfulness of both the ones submitting requests, and those doing the praying. There were many testimonies given by prayer team members on the profound ways they themselves experienced personal spiritual growth and closeness to God by participating in this ministry. That is the awesome thing about prayer. As we reach outward to serve others, devoting time and mental energy to think and pray about their needs, we receive inward perspective of our own life circumstances. Our faith is increased.

Although intercession is not one of my spiritual gifts, I felt called to accept an invitation last spring to join a small group of women to pray weekly for our children, husbands, and each other. Participating in this group helped me discover practical benefits of Connection and Direction in an area of my spiritual life that was incomplete and immature:

- Fellowship – I made new friends. Our friendship is genuine, because it is our common love of the Lord and doing His work together that binds us. In sharing our joys and concerns about family members, we have grown beyond superficial, casual friendship to an intimate knowledge of one another and the people we cherish. We love each other.

- Mentoring – Our leader and hostess showed me how to integrate prayer into my daily routine in a very practical and easy way. No issue or concern is too small for us to place before the group for prayer – a husband's business meeting, or a child's doctor visit. She taught us to release our false modesty and agree that waiting until we meet

75

is not a requirement! It only takes a few seconds to broadcast a short text message describing a prayer need to each other by phone.

- Discipline – In addition to our weekly prayer sessions together, I found time during the week to review our list and continue to seek God on behalf of these ladies and their families. I am now more likely to pause and pray for my own normal events and decisions throughout the day – truly the essence of Higher Choices.

- Encouragement – Because others were aware of our personal goals, we were encouraged when they asked, "How's it going?" We prayed for one another to receive God's guidance and inspiration in the pursuit of goals. This whole process reminded each to remain focused on the goal, and to keep working.

- Peace – We are not meant to carry our burdens alone. 1Peter 5:7 tells us, *"Casting the whole of your care [all your anxieties, all your worries, all your concerns, once and for all] on Him, for He cares for you affectionately and cares about you watchfully."* Allowing others to pray for you helps you release your worries. God wants to carry your burden and give you peace. Trusted prayer partners are a vital part of fully releasing the burden as well.

Take time to seek the Lord on behalf of friends and family. Ask God to guide and protect your children each day at school. Support your local pastor and church leadership by praying for strength and commitment to God's work. Ask that they continually grow in faith. Pray for your nation's leaders, that they would be wise and act not in their own self-interest, but seek justice and peace for the common good.

It is especially important to pray with positive expectation. The Bible tells us to believe when we ask, and we will receive according to our faith. So thank the Lord in advance for what he is doing in others' lives. Follow the example of your faith ancestors by recalling to God His promises in the Word, knowing He is faithful.

Exploration: Be intentional about praying for others.

1. List some promises of God. Identify a person who especially needs to realize each of these promises, and say a prayer for them.

2. Record known prayer requests and subsequent answers (as made known to you) in a journal to both remember to pray frequently, and see how God is moving in the lives of your friends and family.

3. Do you feel a prompting to lift up a particular person in prayer this week?

4. What has been your experience with intercessory prayer? How would you like to grow in this discipline?

> Pray at all times (on every occasion, in every season) in the Spirit, with all [manner of] prayer and entreaty. To that end keep alert and watch with strong purpose and perseverance, interceding in behalf of all the saints (God's consecrated people).
> – Ephesians 6:18 (AMP)

Turning Point 4 – Worship

Holy, holy, holy, Lord God Almighty! Early in
the morning our song shall rise to thee.
– Reginald Heber

Objective: Exalt and worship the Lord in word and song.

Position: There are aspects of prayer that are forms of worship, and aspects of worship that are forms of prayer. Worship is defined as, "reverent honor and homage paid to God or a sacred personage," and "to feel an adoring reverence or regard for." One synonym for worship is "exalt". When the psalmist says, "*Bless the name of the Lord*," he means to extol as holy or to glorify. Thus, you can see that the Adoration component of the A.C.T.S. acrostic directs you to remember that God's holiness, righteousness, compassion, and faithfulness are worthy of your reverence.

In <u>Purpose Driven Life</u>[57], author Rick Warren names worship as one of the believer's main purposes. He says that it is our "number one priority on earth." We experience worship in the church in many forms. Regardless of the style, e.g., formal, contemporary, or blended, a church's order of worship usually includes time for both individual and corporate prayer. Corporate prayer allows us to benefit from written liturgy and the gifts and experience of the prayer leader, as they guide our hearts to specific places for specific reasons. It may be a simple paragraph like this one from <u>A Guide To Prayer For All God's People</u>[63], which says, "Merciful God, were it not for your mercy, I would remain lost in sin and confusion. Thank you for your extravagant grace and your mercy without limit. In this hour hold me in love, even as a mother cradles her child. Amen." Then, we begin to bring what we learn in worship into our individual prayer conversations.

Additionally, hymns, praise songs, anthems, and doxologies can be types of prayers. Music enhances prayer by engaging our emotions, enabling us to express through music what words alone cannot. Often the melody lingers in our minds long after the singing has stopped, and aids us in continuous prayer as the day progresses. Many of the Psalms are prayers, and written as songs to be sung by the people. One of my favorite choral works is John Rutter's Requiem[40]. The second movement is based upon Psalm 130, a Song of Ascent. Verse 1 begins, *"Out of the depths I cry to you, O Lord; O Lord hear my voice."* Continuing with verse 7, *"O Israel, put your hope in the Lord, for with the Lord is unfailing love and with him is full redemption."* You cannot listen to this piece of music and not be inspired to agree with the psalmist and pray these prayers also.

True worship is not a spectator event, but an encounter with the living God. Come before the Lord in an attitude of awe and wonder, and He will meet you there. Jack Hayford, in Worship His Majesty[25], says, "Worship has the power to penetrate hearts, for the child like beauty and authenticity of true worship bypasses resistant minds and touches souls with the tender reality of God's Presence." God is surely always present in any and all forms of your private conversational, intercessory prayer, and meditation, but worship reminds us of who He is, so His presence is recognized as His grace in action.

Not long ago I experienced an evening where I felt a strange concoction of emotions - sadness and fear, mixed with extreme gratitude and hopefulness. The sadness and fear came from the uncertainty, pain, and disillusionment of a personal trial I was going through. The extreme gratitude and hopefulness came from seeing clearly how God had surrounded me with wonderful friends to offer support, comfort, prayer, and concern, despite the fact that most were not even aware of the nature of my ordeal. Fortunately, the happier emotions were the stronger ones. I felt prompted, in a way I never had before, to set aside the majority of the next day for personal worship. I wanted to draw near to God to express my thankfulness in praise, and I needed to feel God's comforting arms around me, and hear his words of assurance. So, I made a little plan. I had early morning quiet time with some Bible study as usual. I ate a light breakfast, and then put on praise music while I cleaned the kitchen and completed some minor chores around the apartment. During a particularly meaningful, favorite songs, I stopped to sit and sing along, offering true praise to my Lord. Following that, I worked through my solitary yoga routine, which is a form of meditation for me. It calms my mind and increases my mental focus. Next on the worship plan, was playing the piano. I played and sang classical pieces, hymns, and praise songs for about one hour. I ended with a little guitar practice. I closed my worship with prayer. Just now, as I read what I wrote in my Prayer Journal that day, I can reconnect with God, feeling again the "overwhelming flood of your love through my friends," and saying, "Thank you! I feel like you are reassuring me, telling me you are working on my behalf."

Enrich and strengthen your prayer life through regular worship participation. Notice that I did not use the word "attendance." It is your participation that makes it true worship.

Exploration: Discover the special ways you connect to God through worship.

1. Public worship: Attend one or more church worship services.

2. Private worship: Set aside 30 minutes to an hour. Select one word of adoration that begins with each letter of

the alphabet to exalt the Lord, all the way from A to Z. For example: Awesome, Beautiful, Caring, Dependable, etc.

3. What component of corporate and private worship touches your heart the most?

4. In what ways do you experience God's presence? What does it feel like?

A man can no more diminish God's glory by refusing to worship Him than a lunatic can put out the sun by scribbling the word, 'darkness' on the walls of his cell.
– C.S. Lewis

DESTINATION

Man is asked to make himself what he is
supposed to become to fulfill his destiny.
— Paul Tillich

Orientation 5 - Fulfill God's purpose for your life by discovering your gifts and passion.

We all want a successful life, but how do we know when we have achieved it? Success is such a subjective term. It means different things to different people. Can you clearly and specifically describe what success means to you? A person seeking to make Higher Choices agrees that their God-given purpose is the path to their most successful life.

What do you think Jesus meant when he said, *"I came that you may have life, and have it abundantly"* (John 10:10)? Abundance is "an extremely plentiful or oversufficient quantity or supply: overflowing fullness; affluence; wealth." Success, on the other hand, is defined as "the favorable or prosperous termination of attempts or endeavors; the attainment of wealth, position, honors, or the like; a successful performance or achievement." What is the difference between abundance and success, and is that important? My observation is that Jesus makes a distinction between what the world considers success, namely status and achievement for personal gain, and what the Father intends as true fulfillment and affluence. The motivation behind our efforts separates abundance from success. The phase "overflowing fullness" conjures an image of abundance as clear, fresh water springing up and over from the inside. Conversely, success seems more like a cup of water sought and drawn from the well outside. Yet, as with many paradoxes in God's kingdom, seeking Him as the path to abundance also leads to success.

Abundant life is a function of your receptiveness to your God-capacity. It is a life lived on purpose, fueled by a passion to express yourself in love and service, and the satisfaction of knowing you make a difference. Your purpose is unique. The combination of your gifts, talents, heritage, experience, personality, and desires are like no one else's. Fulfilling your God-capacity is fulfilling your destiny, and to know your Destination, you have to know yourself. What do you desire and what are you passionate about?

The four Turning Points you will consider in this orientation are:

1. Spiritual Gifts - The things you love to do, and do well, make you an important and unique instrument in God's kingdom.

2. Values & Beliefs - Clarify your values and beliefs, recognizing them as key drivers of your priorities and choices.

3. Mission – Your mission affirms you identity and function from God's perspective.

4. Vision – Paint a mental image of your ideal life, believing God inspires it.

Get to know yourself from God's perspective. Find out what brings you joy, why you make the decisions and choices you do right now, and how to turn those into Higher Choices. Learn the power of formulating a written statement to remind yourself who you are, and how that leads to truly abundant life. Warning: This journey requires effort! However, unlike the thousands of hours people squander in pursuit of success, your work will be rewarded by the source of abundance revealed deep within.

TURNING POINT 1 – SPIRITUAL GIFTS

*Mature believers do not remain independent of
others - rather, they offer their uniqueness to others
and receive from others their differences.*
– Bruce Bugbee & Don Cousins

Objective: The things you love to do, and do well, make you an important and unique instrument in God's kingdom.

Position: "You do not see the significance of who you are." Former Girl Scout CEO, Francis Hesselbein, quoted these words of Peter Drucker at a Geneva College leadership seminar I attended. Upon hearing this quote, my immediate thought was "yes," thinking about how many people I know who fail to realize what they have to offer. You do not have to be in charge of a business or service group to be a leader. People who know their purpose and destination are leaders, because they demonstrate the abundance gained in a life of fulfilling service. Leaders take initiative.

Ms. Hesselbein co-authored a very fine book entitled, <u>Be * Know * Do. Leadership the Army Way</u>[26], which describes the order of a leader's priorities. She writes, "There are three aspects to leadership regardless of organizational level or military rank: who you are inside, what you know, and how you act." I think these are also God's priorities for us. We are to *be* the person God intends, *know* our callings and be competent, and then *do* the work set before us. You must be comfortable with who you are, and "be," before you set about doing. Understanding your spiritual gifts is fundamental to knowing who God calls you to be, as are your values(covered in the next Turning Point). God loves His children so much that each one is uniquely gifted to be a special person contributing to God's plan for the world. Spiritual gifts define your role in God's kingdom. Embracing this idea is a key step in discerning your Higher Choices, because once you know your purpose, Higher Choices are easily recognized.

Sometimes discovering your gifts will not be a surprise. They will be similar and complimentary to natural skills or interests you have had all along. However, they are not the same as natural talents. The resource I use in teaching spiritual gifts is <u>Network: The Right People, in the Right Place, at the Right Time, for the Right Reason</u>[7]. Not only do Bugsby and Cousins describe a large number of spiritual gifts (23), ensuring that all believers can connect with at least one in the assessment, but they help us see how the unique combination of a person's spiritual gifts, personality, and passion amalgamate to embody the concept "be." Two people can share a set of spiritual gifts, yet because one prefers to work with people, particularly one-one-one, and the other is motivated by having a task to accomplish, they will extend their gifts in different ways. Add to that the other dimensions of their heart's passion, personal experience, and present circumstances, and you can see the importance of this personal knowledge as a prerequisite for making Higher Choices about what to "do," when, where, and why.

I had the pleasure of teaching a six-week spiritual gifts class to my Kuala Lumpur Bible study group. It is thrilling and fulfilling for me to see women come alive, to sparkle with enthusiasm and confidence when they realize their passion serves God and serves others. They feel affirmed, because it turns out that what they thought was just a hobby is indeed a service others need. They feel confident, because they see that the Holy Spirit equips, enables, and sustains them when they use their gifts. Alex is a prime example. She displayed keen interest in the details of all our Bible lessons. She passionately participated in our discussions, usually sitting quietly to absorb all that was being said, and then challenging the group with probing questions. In casual conversation, Alex mentioned that she often spent time at the local coffee shop with her friends – my, how the time would fly during those chats. When Alex discovered that her highest spiritual gift is evangelism, the whole group could see her face light up with recognition and relief. She saw that her passion for understanding the Word, combined with her love of connecting with other women one-to-one, enabled her to be an evangelist in her own special way. Knowing her spiritual gifts relieved her from trying to think up ways to serve God, and gave her the confidence to be intentional about sharing the Lord in simple conversation over coffee.

Although a spiritual gift may be similar to natural abilities, awareness of your spiritual gifts will reveal untapped sources of enjoyment, and open doors to new adventures. God's ways usually are not what we expect. Many feel called into some form of ministry or new business venture before the required talents and skills are mature. To me, this is a distinguishing feature of spiritual gifts. It is a blessing in disguise. When we feel inadequate, we are forced to A.S.K. - Ask for God's guidance, Seek God's ideas, Knock against obstacles, and Abide in the Lord, trusting in His plan for how it will all work out. As you follow this process, the peace and joy of knowing who you are helps you relax into "being," trusting that the "doing" will come through the Spirit.

Inspiration and innovation culminate as you use your gifts alongside others, exchanging new ideas and insights, strategies and accomplishments. This is part of what Bugsby and Cousins call interdependence. "That is the way God intends the church to function. Believers come together by serving with their Spiritual Gifts – each doing their part creating something they could never accomplish on their own – the fullness of Christ is revealed." Embracing your spiritual gifts is not only a source of confidence, inspiration, and innovation, but freedom as well. You have the freedom to say "yes" or "no" to opportunities that do or do not involve your gifts. You have confidence to explore new ways to apply your gifts and talents, because you will feel God's blessing and support.

Exploration: Discover and embrace your spiritual gifts as the map to your Destination.

1. Discover your spiritual gifts. Consult one or more of the many spiritual gift inventories available. Ask two or three friends or family members what gifts they see in you.

2. Think of ways you have served others in the past and felt especially connected and fulfilled. List the type of group(s) and activities performed.

3. If you know your spiritual gifts, how are you using them now?

4. If one of your gifts is in an area somewhat new to you, how can you begin to "know" more about it?

*We have many parts in the one body, and all these parts
have different functions. So we are to use our different
gifts in accordance with the grace that God has given us.
– Romans 12:4, 6 (GNB)*

Turning Point 2 – Values & Beliefs

*There's no place else to turn but inward,
to the self, as the locus of values.*
– Abraham H. Maslow

Objective: Clarify your values and beliefs, recognizing them as key drivers of your priorities and choices.

Position: Tony Robbins was the first person to impress upon me the significant role my values and beliefs play in determining my actions. Values drive actions, by driving choices. Tony portrays the tie between values and beliefs with the image of a table, where the top is the value, supported by the legs, which are the beliefs. What you and I believe about something will determine its value to us. Picture yourself standing on top of your value table. What are you standing for? Is it supporting your dreams and releasing your God-capacity?

People share common values, but grant them varying degrees of precedence. Even if two people agree on values and their ranking, their beliefs about a particular value may vary. You and your best friend may both value money, but your respective definitions or interpretations of that may differ. For example, if I believe that money is only one of my resources, of which God calls me to be a good steward, then I will do what I can to live a good life with adequate resources. Conversely, if I believe money can buy everything, then making money will consume my every ounce of energy I have.

Stating your belief about something clarifies its meaning. You may not even realize what you value until you take time to think about them and write them down. A values clarification statement literally allows your values to be seen, and helps you understand why you make the choices you do. A two or three sentence description of your values helps your mind create an image of the associated behavior or action. This image allows you and others to see and recognize it. The beliefs you hold about each value are revealed by your clarification statement.

Knowing your Destination requires that you know your passion. Your most cherished, "core[30]" value is often the best representation of your passion, the best way to describe it, because it is the essence of who you are. Identifying it can be challenging, but there are a couple of questions you can ask yourself: 1) what wrong would you like to right?, and 2) what "gift" do you want to give the people with whom you come in contact? It may take some time to discover, but when you do, you will know it and so will others. I had a coaching client who, after working with me on her mission statement, said her core value is grace. As soon as she said it, I smiled and replied, "Yes you are!" She exudes grace in all she does. It is what she wants to be about; it is her gift to all the people she encounters. Now that she is aware of that, and claims that, she can remind herself to "be grace" and she will be living on purpose. It is relevant and applicable at work, home, and in community.

Your values and beliefs drive your life choices, whether consciously or unconsciously. Listing a handful of your top values increases your ability to make choices consistent with those values. You will learn more about the importance of making choices consistent with your values in the Priority Orientation. For now, to discover your purpose, focus on defining your top values and designating one of those as your core value.

Making Higher Choices may involve adopting higher values. As I mentioned before, writing your values on paper will clarify them for you. The A.S.K. process will help you. Ask God to be present during your values review, and guide you toward those that are particularly relevant to your life. If you are honest with yourself, you may change your mind about your current values, and adopt new ones.

Exploration: Discover the driving force behind many of your decisions by identifying your top life values.

1. Review the List of Values (see Appendix) and select your top 5 personal values. Select one and write a clarifying statement for it.

    Example 1: Gratitude – I am thankful for every good gift God gives to me. I trust in His wisdom and love, thus I am open to receive and celebrate whatever comes into my life. "Thanksgiving always precedes the miracle (Ann Voskamp)."

    Example 2: Selfless Service – Put the welfare of the nation, the Army, and subordinates before your own. Selfless service does not mean that a soldier can't have a strong ego, high self-esteem, or even healthy ambition. Rather, selfless service means not making decisions or taking actions that help one's image or one's career but hurts others or sabotages the mission.[26]

2. Are there traits you see in people you admire that may be potential values for you to adopt?

3. Which of the values listed above is the most important? Try "being" that value. How does it cause you to make Higher Choices?

If you must tell me your opinions,
tell me what you believe in.
I have plenty of doubts of my own.
— Johann Goethe

TURNING POINT 3 – MISSION

You are either living your mission or somebody else's.
Which will it be?
– Laurie Beth Jones

Objective: Your mission affirms your identity and function from God's perspective.

Position: I am most grateful for the "God-incident" that brought Laurie Beth Jones into my life. All of her books excellently promote one's connection to "the Divine," but her second book, The Path, Creating Your Mission Statement for Work and for Life[30], is *the* definitive resource for understanding and living your godly purpose. Laurie's inspired approach explains what mission is, and what it is not.

Although many organizations draft mission/vision statements, mission and vision are different. A good mission statement is short. Once clearly defined, it will not change. Contrarily, a vision statement is long. It is a detailed description of the results of you living the mission. Your mission encompasses your entire life, so it enfolds your personal, family, community, and church life, as well as your vocation. You are fulfilling your purpose when you embrace who you are as God's beloved, unique child, and because of this perspective, joyfully and boldly take action to live your passion.

Another distinction between mission and vision is that mission is process. Spiritual gifts, values, and beliefs tell you who to "be."

Mission helps you know what to "do." The key to enjoying life is to enjoy every moment. Clearly, you will only actively continue to do something you love. Spending the majority of your time using your spiritual gifts, consistent with your values, is where you personal joy lies. That is how you experience an abundant, adventurous life.

Serving in music ministry requires many hours of study and practice. I love to practice piano, voice, and guitar. I easily get lost in the music, thinking about what I can learn and improve, that the time just whizzes by! I could just practice classical and pop music, and I do enjoy that. However, my passion for hymns and praise music, combined with my desire to serve the community as a worship leader, makes the process of working on those pieces most fulfilling. When I served as a children's choir director, I enjoyed selecting anthems, deciding how to teach each piece, and planning rehearsals to keep the boys engaged. Likewise, writing and speaking on spiritual formation has the same effect. I enjoy using my gifts of faith and wisdom as I study The Bible, research related topics, work through an inspired idea, and then write and speak about it. The process itself is fulfilling.

So, contrary to what you may have perceived, living your mission will energize you, not wear you out! It is something you easily embrace, not dread. When you live "on purpose," what you do does not feel like work most of the time. What could you do all day without fatigue? What are the most rewarding activities you have undertaken? When do you get lost in time, so the speak?

As Laurie says, "A mission statement truly is like a harness and a sword, because it harnesses you to what it true, and cuts away all that is false." Once you discover your mission, you will most likely have to "cut away" something that no longer serves you or anyone else. Staying on mission means that you will continue on your right path, aligned with True North, ready for whatever adventure awaits around the next turn.

Exploration: Spend time discovering your mission. It is fundamental to living God's call on your life.

1. What activity engages you for long periods, where you do not think about time?

2. What is your core value? What do you want to give to those you love and serve?

3. What false beliefs and actions do you need to cut away to make room for your true mission?

4. Write a one-sentence statement that combines your spiritual gifts in action with your core value.

   a. Example: I inspire, demonstrate and promote vision, and the possibilities of purposeful living.

   b. Example: I encourage and support co-workers and family through my gracious attitude, communication, and demeanor.

> When I become my dreams, I live to the
> rhythm of the Divine reason for my life.
> When I don't, my soul is painfully silent.
> – Karyn D. Kedar

TURNING POINT 4 – VISION

The doors that bar us from our dreams are imaginary. If you do not see them, you will walk right through them.
-- Karyn D. Kedar

Objective: Paint a mental picture of your ideal life, believing God inspires it.

Position: Do you have a favorite post card or photo from a memorable trip? Do you have a painting you love to gaze at, one that simply makes you smile? Perhaps you have viewed a landscape scene that made you wish you could jump right into to experience it for yourself. Images powerfully engage your mind. To reach your Destination you need to picture a place that captivates you. A vision statement is a word picture of your ideal life. The power of having a personal vision statement is that it engages both your mental vision, and the emotions you attach to that. As you focus on your vision, you will be motivated to do what is necessary to bring it into your life. And when you experience days when your mission does seem a bit onerous, your vision statement will re-energize you to keep moving.

Johnny Cash was an inspiring man who, despite traveling the rough and rocky road of addition, touched many lives by remaining faithful to his passion for the Lord, and helping the less fortunate. I do not think Cash had a crystallized vision of his life's destiny, however his contributions indicate he was compelled by a dream to share his music and other talents, shining his light so others might see God, and experience a better life. He had an initial vision of himself as a Gospel musician. He was that, and much more. Cash "made a spoken word recording of the entire New King James Version of the New Testament. Even so, Cash declared that he was 'the biggest sinner of them all', and viewed himself overall as a complicated and contradictory man.[44]" He had purpose and imagination in his decision to dress in black for all of his performances. "In 1971, Cash wrote the song 'Man in Black', to help explain his dress code: 'We're doing mighty fine I do suppose / In our streak of lightning cars and fancy clothes / But just so we're reminded of the ones who are held back / Up front there ought to be a man in black.' He wore black on behalf of the poor and hungry, on behalf of 'the prisoner who has long paid for his crime,' and on behalf of those who have been betrayed by age or drugs. [44]" Cash worked with many music legends, starred in television and film, and met with the President of the United States. It seems to me that Johnny Cash was successful, because he embraced his gifts, took action to promote his godly passion, and imagined that life for his fellow man, family, and himself would benefit from it. He experienced many bad days, but did not let the dream die.

Not every vision equates to success. Too many people sacrifice inner peace and personal happiness in their pursuit of material success. When your life vision merges with God's you seek abundance, and success follows. Earlier I contrasted abundance and success. True success is a combination of prosperity, fulfillment, happiness, and peace. God blesses effort exerted for the sake of your mission, because you will bring glory to His name. Your Destination is the picture of the life that pleases both you and God. It is possible to have the desires of your heart and be obedient at the same time! In fact, none of us can even imagine the good God wants to bring into our lives. Psalm 37:4 says, *"Delight yourself in the Lord and he will give you the desires of your heart."* The book of Isaiah contains many verses that describe God's vision for the people, such as *"They will feed beside the roads and find pasture on every barren hill. They will neither hunger nor thirst, nor will the desert heat or the sun beat upon them"* (Isaiah 49:9-10).

Give yourself permission to dream while you A.S.K. to discover what God's vision for you might be. You cannot create a beautiful life if you do not know what it should look like. Spend quality, prayerful time imaging what you would like to experience, where you would like to go, and whom you would like to spend time with. Cast a vision of what life will look like one to three years from now – the result of you living your mission. Your values clarification statements are actually small snapshots that form pieces of your larger vision. Include the various roles you currently have, and any new ones you would like to create. Here are a few "images" taken from my personal vision statement:

- Coaching – It is such a thrill to meet with my coaching clients and help them discover their path. I conduct both individual and group coaching sessions, on the phone, over the internet, and in person. I speak regularly at group events, and deliver workshops every quarter. The time I spend in research and writing is also enjoyable. I am well compensated for my work.

- Fitness – I lovingly care for my body, and in return, have an abundance of energy to accomplish all of my goals. Running and yoga keep me fit; it is a great way to start my day. I enjoy cooking healthy recipes, and sharing them with friends and family. Physical fitness improves my mental, emotional, and spiritual attitudes.

Because God is the god, *"... who is able to do immeasurably more than all we ask or imagine..."* (Ephesians 4:20), trust that as you have worked through all of the Explorations in this orientation, the resulting combined image will lead you to your Destination.

Exploration: Ask God to give you a detailed vision, and write it down.

1. How clearly and specifically can you describe what success looks like to you?

2. Are you "seeing" glimpses of a new Destination? What part of your vision can you start living today?

3. What would you do if you knew you could not fail?

4. Set aside one hour. With your values clarification statements in hand, write a two to three page detailed description of your ideal life. Where are you? Who are you with? What are you doing during the week and on the weekends? Be sure to include descriptive adjectives to make it engaging.

Except the Lord builds the house, they labor in vain who build it; except the Lord keeps the city, the watchman wakes but in vain.

> It is vain for you to rise up early, to take rest
> late, to eat the bread of [anxious] toil – for He
> gives [blessing] to His beloved in sleep.
> – Psalm 127:1-2 (AMP)

COURSE

*Guide me, O thou great Jehovah, pilgrim through
this barren land. I am weak, but thou art
mighty; hold me with thy powerful hand.*
— William Williams

**Orientation 6 - You will not arrive at your Destination
by accident. You must chart the Course.**
Working through the Exploration questions and exercises to discover
your Destination is a tremendous accomplishment. Congratulations.
I hope you feel good about yourself, and possess a keen motivation
to move toward it. Now you begin to turn your vision into reality.
You need a solid plan to embark on your new adventure. Charting
the course is a critical skill and discipline most people skip, and
then wonder why their life does not turn out the way they thought
it would.

Whether or not you are a good planner, following the principles in
this Orientation will increase the likelihood that your Course is clear
and manageable.

The four Turning Points you will consider in this orientation are:

1. Goals - Set goals as intermediate arrival points that
   allow you to realize your vision in mini adventures

2. Resources - Identify the time, material, financial, and human resources you will need, and who can supply them.

3. Speed - Relax your travel speed to allow for changing objectives and circumstances. Enjoy the journey.

4. Productivity - Establish a personal productivity system you can trust to keep you on Course.

Mission and vision statements are essential for defining your purpose, your Destination. Charting the Course leads you through the process of defining specific goals, that when accomplished, result in small images that will allow you to see your vision take shape. What will you need to accomplish your goals? You will need time (aren't you busy enough already!), money, and help from other people. Personal organization plays an important role in planning. In this chapter, you will evaluate your current productivity system to see if it is adequate for creating a reliable, flexible map you will depend upon. Be diligent in your work to put serious detail into your life's plan. You will recoup the time spent by experiencing peaceful productivity. Let God guide your efforts so you can enjoy the adventure together.

TURNING POINT 1 – GOALS

The best way to predict the future is to create it.
– Peter Drucker

Objective: Set goals as intermediate arrival points that allow you to realize your vision in mini adventures.

Position: Setting goals leads you to your Destination by breaking the Course down into manageable sojourns. Charting the Course is like mapping out any travel plan. Identify and include checkpoints and rest stops to make the journey stimulating.

Think of your vision as a puzzle, where goals are the puzzle pieces. Accomplishing a goal produces a tangible picture that represents part of your ideal life. As the pieces take shape and you see how they fit together, you will be inspired to continue on the adventure, anticipating the complete picture.

I saw a child's rendering of a mountain landscape taped to the doctor's office cabinet above the checkout clerk recently. It reminded me of the way I drew, repeatedly, a favorite landscape picture as a child. I started with two curved lines to form the rolling hills, adding cloud-like puffs on top of stilts for trees, a semi-circle with radiating lines in the corner for the sun, and pairs of tiny convex lines for the birds in the sky flying lazily over the meadow. I drew one thing at time, perhaps beginning with the sun, or maybe the meadow. Once I finished that, I moved on to add more interesting characters and sites. The picture came alive, became what I willed it to be, as each elementary stroke left its mark and inspired me to make another.

Setting goals may sound boring, but actually, it is very motivating. Goals are not the same as a task list! Goals should be *SMART: Specific, Measurable, Attainable, Relevant, and Time-bound*[39]. Stating that you want to develop a children's ministry is not a goal. It is the beginning of a vision. It is a lovely part of your vision, but that broad statement is not specific enough to give direction. What will the children do or learn? How are you specifically using your gifts in this ministry? What is God showing you the children need? These types of questions (Ask) foster the ideas (Seek) that can be stated as goals. Get started by defining one important goal. For example, you may need to gather more information to answer the questions above, in which case your first goal might be to meet with the Children's Coordinator of your church to share your ideas and brainstorm. Setting a goal to meet with this person is specific, attainable, and relevant. For it to be measurable, it must answer the question "When am I done?" or "What is the tangible evidence the task has been completed?" The results of your discussions with the Children's Coordinator, e.g., your meeting notes and follow up action items, are evidence the goal has been achieved. Your goal must also have a due date. The average person has a mediocre life because they skip this critical step. If you do not set a target completion date, you will easily let it be forgotten and never accomplished.

Define a goal from each meaningful paragraph in your vision statement and each value clarification statement. This will ensure that you are progressing in all areas of your life. Many goals involve multiple tasks or action steps, so you will want to set both long-term and short-term goals. List and order all the steps you can, and give each a due date. This is a living, flexible plan, so if you are not sure of the dates, select them as best you can (more on this in the

Speed Turning Point). The dates can be revised as more information becomes available.

Begin today! As the picture takes shape, you will be inspired to add more. You will love what you see, and experience the elation of creating something uniquely yours.

Exploration: Break your Destination down into manageable treks by creating long-range and short-term goals.

1. Can you remember a goal you accomplished in the past? How did it feel? What goal(s) can you set today to get that feeling again?

2. Setting goals provides structure for the Seek step of the A.S.K. process. Which goal or goals can you put on your calendar this week, this month, and this year?

3. Divide your vision statement into categories by role, value, or activity type. You will have a paragraph length description to narrow your focus.

   Example: Music Vision - I regularly serve as a worship leader. I design the worship format and liturgical content for weekly worship events. I combine my music and coaching talents to offer uniquely spiritually engaging workshops and retreats. The traditional hymns and Taize' music I love makes my style appealing to a wide variety of seekers and faithful worshipers. I am an accomplished, self-accompanied singer, using both guitar and piano, and enjoy practicing both instruments five times each week.

4. For each category list all goals that come to mind, checking to ensure they are SMART. Designate a due date now. You may change it later. Selecting a target

date of 3 or 6 months into the future is a good way to start.

Example: Music Goals

• Learn 2 classical piano pieces each month

• Learn 2 hymns each month with piano accompaniment

• Design the worship music weekend retreat by June 1st.

• Design Taize' worship service with instrumentation by November 30th.

5. Many goals must be broken down into smaller action steps. List all the steps you can currently identify for each goal. Arrange them in the order to be completed where applicable.

To will is to select a goal, determine a course of action that will bring one to that goal, and then hold to that action til the goal is reached. The key is action.
– Michael Hanson

Turning Point 2 – Resources

*We don't accomplish anything in this world alone
... and whatever happens is the result of the whole
tapestry of one's life and all the weavings of individual
threads from one to another that creates something.*
– Sandra Day O'Connor

Objective: Identify the time, material, financial, and human resources you will need, and who can supply them.

Position: I have forgotten exactly who told me you have to spend money to make money, but I have found that principle to be true. That phrase tells me every worthwhile thing has a cost. Some form of resources will be required to accomplish your goals and stay on Course. You have probably already guessed what your key resources are, especially if you served any time in the corporate world: *Time, Money, and People.*

Remember that a principle benefit of Higher Choices is Connection and Direction. Connecting with people is the most important thing. Who is currently working with or around the people who will be served by you living your mission? How do your goals assist them, or compliment their endeavors? What's in it for them? Begin to establish your network by identifying and approaching these folks. Not only can they supply key material resources, but they can also lend support, guidance, and encouragement. As you connect with others in your areas of interest, they will affect your direction and you will influence theirs.

My first thought about how to chart a course to get more involved in the church music program was to share my goal with our church music minister. I trusted her to be receptive and kind when I expressed my desire to fulfill part of my purpose. Perhaps, I thought, she would also be willing to give her advice. I surmised she would welcome enthusiastic and committed volunteer help, because I had the potential to be a resource for her goals! "The rest is history," as the saying goes. I started helping with the boy choir, and for the next several years, continued to learn, grow, and achieve many goals through this friend, teacher, and encourager.

Money is also needed to achieve most goals. You may have some of the money, but not all of it. Many times, the same people you will be working with can help supply the money as well. In the Progress Orientation we will discuss your responsibility to develop and expand your gifts. Thus, one of your goals may be to take a class, attend a workshop, or buy some equipment. Over the years I have spent money on piano, guitar, and voice lessons, a piano, a guitar, music books, website development, printing, travel…you get the idea.

Time seems to be the scarcest resource. We do not really manage time; we manage events and commitments. You will focus more on how to maximize your time in the Speed Turning Point and the Priority Orientation. For now, just estimate the time required, and prepare yourself to commit that to achieve your goals.

God provides. Co-creating your life through Higher Choices means that God is with you every step of the way, supplying your every need. Trust that what you need will be available when you need it. We can create havoc in our lives when we step out of God's provision and try to manifest "things" before their time. Be diligent in identifying, securing, and appropriating necessary resources, and then "just do it." The next required allotment of time, money, or whatever will appear if you stay true to your Course.

Exploration: List the required resources for the goals you have identified.

1. Who would love to help you achieve your goals? Who will you be serving by living your mission?

2. What material resources do you have, and what do you need to acquire? Can you spend money you have now more wisely to reach your dreams?

3. How can you structure your regular weekly plan to spend more time on purpose? What are you doing to take advantage of pockets of time that become available?

4. People – List the names of specific persons you would like to meet, and groups you would like to join in your adventure. Identify whether they are a critical resource, or if you can achieve the goal without them.

   Example:
   Goal – Design Taize' Worship with Instrumentation.
   Myself
   Experienced Taize' Worship Leader for consultation
   Worship Sponsor

5. Money – List all material resources required to for each goal, including supplies and funds required to pay for services. Indicate whether the material resources are currently available, or must be required. Estimate the cost of each item.

   Example:
   Goal – Design Taize' Worship with Instrumentation.

Taize' references including print music ($0 - available)
Sample Taize' recorded music ($45)
Notebook or binder with paper ($10)
Experienced Taize' Worship Consultant ($80)
Worship Sponsor ($0)
Myself ($0)

6. Time – Estimate the total time, in hours, required for each human resources listed above.

Example:
Goal – Design Taize' Worship with Instrumentation.
Experienced Taize' Worship Consultant (2 hr)
Worship Sponsor (2 hr)
Myself (15 hr)

Never forget the three powerful resources you always have available to you: love, prayer, and forgiveness.
– H. Jackson Brown, Jr.

Turning Point 3 – Speed

*Half our life is spent trying to find something to do with
the time we have rushed through life trying to save.*
– Will Rogers

Objective: Relax your travel speed to allow for changing objectives
and circumstances. Enjoy the journey.

Position: Process rules! This is the most important principle to keep
in mind as you chart the Course. You are supposed to enjoy the
adventure of what you are doing, while you are doing it. Trying
to accomplish goals too fast is a sure way to get yourself derailed,
risking a crash into the embankment of accomplishment. You will
get frustrated, stressed out, and likely give up.

The short-term and long-range goals you have set are your checkpoints
along the road to your Destination. Let them serve their purpose
of supplying rest, perspective, assessment, and accomplishment.
Because this is your plan, the pace is largely up to you. You are
the one dictating the route and schedule. You will learn how to
handle the myriad of ways your course will change in the Priorities,
Progress, and Navigation Orientations. The purpose of this Turning
Point is to map the ideal timing, assuming no interruptions.

John Ortberg says, "We must radically eliminate hurry from our
lives.[37]" I have learned this lesson the hard way! I used to be in a
hurry, rarely happy unless I felt I was accomplishing something.
Living in Malaysia helped me follow the advice I give clients to slow

down. My fellow expats and I used to laugh about "Malaysia time," which is akin to "island time." No one is in a hurry to do much of anything, and you can bet whatever you would like to have done is going to take twice as long as you think. Traffic, is a prime example. People will zoom by and cut you off, yet end up waiting right beside you stuck in the same jam!

Life presents you with opportunities. You need to be ready to take advantage of them. You will not be able to, however, if with your schedule overbooked, you are running at full speed with your eyes straight ahead. Not only will the time for action not be available no matter what commitments you alter, neither will you have the presence of mind to notice the opportunities passing you by. You learned earlier that you must remove the static in your life in order to hear and respond to the promptings from the Holy Spirit. Speed is another response inhibitor! If you cannot recognize His cues, your adventure with God will be limited. Traveling fast will get you to where you are heading quickly, but whatever that place is, may not be your true Destination.

Make time to be "on purpose," and enjoy the process. Your mission encompasses all your roles, thus should occupy about 80% of your time. Within each category of activity, schedule enough time to keep your interest and motivation high, without letting it become a burden - something you dread or feel guilty about. God's will is for you to enjoy the journey through peaceful productivity.

Exploration: Map your Course at a pace that allows to you enjoy working toward your goals while being productive.

1. Have you been in too much of a hurry lately? What problems or pain has that caused?

2. If your dream opportunity were available today, would you be ready to seize it?

3. Determine the calendar time available for each goal. Get a monthly calendar covering the next six to twelve months. Record all known commitments and regular engagements to indicate "unavailable" time. Note holidays, vacations, and special days as well.

4. Review your goals and tasks and construct a timeline showing tasks to complete in succession, and those you can be working on simultaneously. Identify points of no action where you may need to wait on someone or something before you can proceed.

5. Overlay the timeline onto the calendar. Adjust goal and task start and end dates to accommodate the time you have available to commit to each activity.

> *Not everything is what is seems to be. Slow down and consider the levels of meaning. These slowed frames are God moments.*
> *– Karyn D. Kedar*

Turning Point 4 – Productivity

There is usually an inverse proportion between how much something is on your mind and how much it's getting done.
– David Allen

Objective: Establish a personal productivity system you can trust to keep you on Course.

Position: The people I know who are living the life they want are organized. No matter his or her personality or preferences, tendencies or style, they have some way of being productive when they have to. Some use email; some use an old-fashioned daily calendar by the phone. Some use a Blackberry®, email inbox, student agenda supplied by the school, or simply Post-It!® notes and slips of paper. I have a friend who calls her home phone to leave herself voice mail reminders!

David Allen has written a very fine book, <u>Getting Things Done</u>³, where he explains that you have to trust your personal productivity system in order for it to be effective. He points out that the main purpose of whatever system you choose is to clear your mind. You do that by recording all your appointments, phone calls, errands, etc. in a place where you will be able to recall quickly what you need, and take the appropriate action. A reliable personal productivity system reduces stress and anxiety. A clear mind is a productive mind.

The instructor who taught the first management training seminar I attended began his presentation by stepping to front center stage holding a large black leather day planner high above his head. With a commanding voice he said, "If you don't have one of these, go get one." He then went on to explain the virtues of a time management system. I have been sort of a day planner junky ever since. The style and size of my system, both hard copy and electronic, has morphed along with job changes and shifting roles and responsibilities. Currently, I use Outlook® to record planned appointments and tasks, and to flag email messages for "Follow Up." It also contains my address book. Every item is assigned to a category, such as Home, Coaching, Church, Kids, Personal, and so on. Color-coding the categories makes them pop on the screen and printed page. I have another software application to organize my tasks into projects. I synchronize all of this with my phone/PDA, because unless you always have it handy, your productivity system will fail you.

It does not matter what system you use. It does matter that you consciously evaluate the effectiveness of your current system, and improve it as you are lead.

Exploration: Declutter your mind of the many "to dos" and appointments you are still trying to store there.

1. Hard copy agendas and electronic organizers both have their pros and cons. Which is best for you, or how can you tailor your own combination?

2. In what ways can you simplify your productivity system, so it does not become another source of tension?

3. Some things you need to accomplish can either be labeled as a Task on your To Do list, or recorded as an appointment. Decide how you want to label each action item in your goals list.

4. Consider how you currently receive, store, and reference email messages and correspondence. Is that working for you?

5. Where do you record general daily or project notes? Are they easily retrievable?

6. Discover the features you like among a variety of planning and productivity systems by visiting your local office supply store, and interviewing your well-organized friends. Try one or two.

Time is what we want most, but what we use worst.
    – William Penn

PRIORITY

He sought God in the days of Zechariah, who had
understanding in the visions of God; and as long
as he sought the Lord, God made him prosper.
– 2 Chronicles 26:5 (NKJ)

Orientation 7 - Realize your "no regrets" life by
making choices consistent with your values.
Everybody has regrets. There are things we wish we had not done, or words we wish we had not said. There are things we should do that we forsake. However, having no regrets is a legitimate goal, because regret is only a feeling we get when we examine the results of our choices. Making Higher Choices leads to fewer regrets.

You have already listed and clarified your values. Whether or not you are conscious of it, whatever you value is naturally, what you will make a priority. This is why clarifying your values are important. We reap what we sow. Are the choices you are making now consistent with your values?

The four Turning Points you will consider in this orientation are:

1.   Observe Priorities – How you spend your most precious resources reveals a great deal about you.

2.   Define Priorities - Making God your highest priority provides time and space for all else to find its place.

115

3. Balance Priorities - Experience God's peace by matching priority choices to short term changes in circumstances.

4. Adjust Priorities - God's purpose for you will take on new dimensions in different seasons of life.

In the Destination Orientation, you combined your mission and highest values to form a vision of the abundant life you will experience fulfilling your call. You set goals and identified the resources you will need in the Course Orientation, and have thus created a high-level plan to live on mission. The best plans are flexible plans. We live in an ever-changing world. You are co-creating with God, which means you have positioned yourself to respond to His leading. Your plan will change! Therefore, you need a framework for making Higher Choices that keeps you on track while maximizing your spontaneity. Defining your priorities builds this framework.

Recall the earlier analogy of the puzzle pieces that come together to create a beautiful picture. If you were to sit at your kitchen table and begin working on a new puzzle, which pieces would you pick up first? Most likely, you would gravitate toward the ones with one or more straight edges. They provide structure for recognizing and assembling the others. Likewise, priorities are boundaries that guide your "being," while the Course guides you "doing." Be, then do. Well defined, balanced priorities guide you to still waters, avoiding the swirling winds of regret.

TURNING POINT 1 – OBSERVE PRIORITIES

I've always thought anyone can make money.
Making a life worth living, that's the real test.
– Robert Fulghum

Objective: How you spend your most precious resources reveals a great deal about you.

Position: I learned from my Walk to Emmaus˚ that you can tell anyone's priorities by where they spend their time and money. This is definitely true! Time and money are your most precious resources. Whether or not you think you can name your priorities, the tell tale signs are all around. Begin by looking at your bank statement and calendar. Your true priorities should be clear. Beyond the obvious resources of time and money, two more priority indicators are: 1) mental focus, and 2) physical energy. What thoughts do you allow to dominate your mind? When you have time to read, what is your choice? What television shows do you watch? Do you exercise and eat well? The answers to these questions reveal your true priorities as well. You can be at home with your family all around you, yet fail to make them a priority if your mind and energy are engrossed by the internet, TV, or the work you brought home.

The dictionary defines a priority as having a state or quality of being earlier in time, order, rank, or privilege. The only way to know the privilege and rank you are granting to anything is to record and analyze some data over time. Your true priorities, as defined by your actions, may not be consistent with the personal image you have of yourself. In my work in software process improvement, I learned there are categories of actions[27]:

- What we ought to do

- What we plan to do

- What we think we do

- What we actually do

I had many software process improvement clients that had to be shown quantitatively that what they planned to do, what they thought they were doing, and what they actually did often were very different. If you visualize each these categories as circles containing all of your actions, to what degree do they overlap? A diagram of the ideal would show only one circle, because each would have the same circumference and position. Perhaps that is not ideal, for it would make for a boring life, not an adventurous one. The point is to know what you actually do, and consider what changes you want to make to better align your actions with your priorities.

Observing your priorities for one week or month will help you know if you are faithful to yourself and your purpose. This is especially important as you work toward replacing some old habits (and goals) with the new ones on your Course. Your personal productivity system is where you can keep a time log to record how you are spending the hours of each day. You planned to work on that design project at least five hours this week. Did you do that? Serving others is one of your values. What exactly did you do for someone this week, and when? In the second Turning Point you will define your priorities. Help yourself make that an effective exercise with real data collection. Once you observe your priorities, the question becomes "Do the priorities observed match what you planned?" "Are your observed priorities Higher Choices?"

The small, seemingly insignificant decisions you make everyday are the tangible steps required to align with True North. Perhaps if the

Pharisees and Scribes had taken time to observe what their words and actions revealed about their commitment to God, they might have been able to see that they were not on Course.

Exploration: Take a thorough inventory of where you spend your time, money, and attention.

1. Keep a time log for one week. A standard weekly calendar works fine. Pause for a few minutes a couple times each day to record what you did. Time increments of 30 to 60 minutes are revealing.

2. Keep a finance log for one week. You may use a sheet of paper, electronic spreadsheet, or the time log. Collect cash receipts. Your bank most likely provides internet access to statements and credit card information. Download a copy for your records.

3. Review both the time and finance log, and divide resources spent by category, e.g., home, kids, leisure, church. Notice your feelings as you review how you actually spent your time and money.

4. If you had a plan for the week, how well did your actual schedule match your plan?

5. What receives the majority of your focus, especially during leisure time? Does that contribute to your energy levels, and mental and emotional states?

6. With whom did you spend the most time? Did you nurture those relationships?

7. What did your log reveal about the priority God receives?

Wherever we are giving our utmost attention, our greatest
gift of time and energy — there will our alter be.
— Laurie Beth Jones

Turning Point 2 – Define Priorities

*The key is not to prioritize what's on your
schedule, but to schedule your priorities.*
– Stephen Covey

Objective: Making God your highest priority provides time and space for all else to find its place.

Position: The most wonderful thing I have learned about seeking to live my purpose, is that God honors my efforts by keeping my resource supply plentiful. The times when I left some things undone done did not matter when I spent time on the top priority areas. Jesus said *"But seek first the kingdom of God and His righteousness, and all these things shall be added to you"* (Matt 6:33 NKJV). Thus, we are to put God first, and everything else will fall into place. The Bible has much to say about the law of sowing and reaping. Thanks to searchable websites offering The Bible online, I found 43 verses containing the word 'sow.' Job 4:8 says, *"As I have seen, those who plow iniquity and sow trouble reap the same"* (ESV). The most memorable, is perhaps the Parable of the Sower, found in Luke chapter 8. Beyond the specific reference to sowing, God's Word clearly tells us that our actions always produce something. We must decide what we are going to produce. Our time, financial, and energy offerings are seeds that grow, yielding a future harvest.

It was in researching the source of my belief about priorities and goals that I was prompted to re-read Stephen R. Covey's <u>The 7</u>

Habits of Highly Effective People[13]. Stephen's work, plus the many years I have used the Franklin Covey organization products, has had a positive influence on me. In the chapter on *Habit 3: Put First Things First*, Stephen poses an important question and challenge to his reader to promote the practice effective self- management. It reads, "Identify a Quadrant II (Important, Not Urgent) activity you know has been neglected in your life – one that, if done well, would have a significant impact in your life, either personally or professionally. Write it down and commit to implement it." I did not have to ponder very long. I knew the one thing I had been neglecting, and that if I recommitted to it, would have a tremendous affect both personally and professionally – consistent prayer and meditation. The answer came so swiftly, it seemed as if the Holy Spirit was sitting right beside me in a classroom, slipping me a note with the test answer written on it! Faithful disciples put God first in their lives. He is their priority. If we trust God to daily guide, protect, and provide, then the most effective thing we can do for ourselves is to give our time and mental focus to God in prayer. Making prayer and meditation a priority does not mean it has to be the first thing done in the morning, although I highly recommend it. It means you do it often and consistently. A discipline like prayer or Bible study is, as Steven writes, important, not urgent. That is why it can be difficult. Email, phone calls and someone else's crisis moment are urgent, because they are noisy. Although I believe prayer is both important and urgent (Quadrant I), it is still too easily pushed to the back burner in today's world where so many things compete for our time and attention.

Spending quiet time with God first thing each morning reminds me that my connection with God is my highest priority. The immediate benefits make the practice easy to maintain. After spending time with God, my priority is to spend time and other resources on those things that are important to God: mission, family, work or school, community, helping others, and enjoying leisure time. Investing in people should be a top priority. I have not always done this, but my relationships receive more focused now.

What did you learn from the Observe Priorities Exploration? What needs to shift? The difficult task for you and I is to eliminate, or at least gradually reduce, those activities that have potential to get us sidetracked. Remember, your priorities drive your decisions. Equipping yourself with a list of your top priorities for each resource will simplify all your decisions, relieve stress, and increase your tendency toward Higher Choices.

Exploration: Rank your new priorities for investing all your resources.

1. List your financial priorities by month and year.

2. List the people and relationships you most treasure and intend to make a priority.

3. It is important to practice good self-care. List your priorities for maintaining health, energy, leisure and self-development.

4. Your Course defines your time management priorities. Review your planned schedule to ensure you are leaving enough time to honor the other priorities you have listed.

5. Is charitable giving included as a financial priority? How much goes toward each goal you set?

6. How are you going to allocate what may seem like small budget of discretionary time? Have you accounted for family, service, and yourself?

7. What printed media, books, audio entertainment, and internet resources are you allowing to feed your mind?

How does this influence your thinking and behavior?
Is it edifying yourself and others?

Decide what you want, decide what you are willing to exchange for it. Establish your priorities and go to work.
— H. L. Hunt

Turning Point 3 – Balance Priorities

*Everyone is crossing the bridge with more weight
than they can handle, so you have to juggle.*
– "God," in Joan of Arcadia

Objective: Experience God's peace by matching priority choices to short term changes in circumstances.

Position: What does it mean to have balance? Balance is a term used to describe a desirable attribute of human life in these recent decades of striving to have it all. We are encouraged to eat balance meals and to balance the checkbook. But how does one obtain balance in life, and why should she care. Balance is synonymous with equilibrium, which the dictionary defines as: 1) bodily balance, 2) emotional stability, 3) situation of balance, and 4) balance between forces. We can gain several insights about balance from all of these definitions. As with bodily balance, life balance requires strength, focus and a sense of our positions relative to the world around us. Describing equilibrium as a "situation" reminds us that balance is a state; a condition that requires our attention and effort to sustain. We all encounter a variety of "forces" at work, home, or in any situation, and it is up to us to choose which ones we move with.

Not long ago I used the gym's Treadclimber˙ for aerobic exercise. This machine had a split treadmill, such that the left and right sides moved in vertical opposition to each other in response to the weight or force I gave it. I found it difficult to keep my balance without holding onto the rail. When I attempted to walk freely, I had to concentrate and focus intently. When I let my mind or eyes wander from my target, I began to stumble. My speed had a great deal to do with it as well. More strength and focus were required to maintain balance at higher speeds.

We feel a sense of life balance in relation to how we spend our time. Time seems to be scarce and largely out of our control. We are out of balance when too much time is devoted to one activity at the expense of another. Scripture tells us *"there is a time for everything, and a season for every activity"* (Ecclesiastes 3:1). Focus on God's priorities for you to achieve your balance. You cannot expect to maintain perfect balance, but you increase in peace and joy when you make Higher Choices concerning the forces you allow to move you. Now that you have defined your priorities, you have built the framework for staying on Course. Yet, it never fails that just as things seem to be going our way, within just in a matter of days some unforeseen circumstance will arise that requires a quick rearrangement of our priorities. That something could be a distraction or an opportunity. Perhaps you have lost focus, or God has something in store for you at these times.

My family loved the Friday night television series Joan of Arcadia[24] that aired a few years ago. As with the historical Joan of Arc, this modern high school teenager is visited by God, who randomly appears in Joan's life as "one of us; just a stranger on the bus," as the theme song says. God, showing up as the lady filling trays in the school cafeteria or the Goth student at his locker, gives Joan seemingly bizarre and always inconvenient assignments. Like a typical seventeen-year-old, Joan feels put out, thus she never sees the significance of her mission until its completion. The humorous, often sarcastic dialogue between God and Joan is priceless! Whatever Joan's priorities may be any given day, they are obliterated when God "drops" into her life. God gives Joan the choice to obey, but at the same time is firm, turning and walking away with a flippant wave "good-bye," indicating that her objections and excuses are useless. Although Joan is helping someone in need and being God's instrument for good, it is Joan who receives the blessings of understanding God more, understanding people more, and being transformed into a young woman who's character becomes more God-like.

Balancing your priorities enables you to stay on purpose across multiple life roles on a consistent basis. Your vocation will consume a large chunk of time, whether or not it is for pay. Family time includes not only spending time with loved ones, but also doing those fun chores like grocery shopping, cooking and cleaning, miscellaneous errands, and appointments. Church and community obligations come and go, nonetheless time must be set aside. So, on one level, you intentionally schedule your time to balance your priorities. On another level, you maintain balance by allowing some slack in your time commitments so you are prepared to handle unforeseen circumstances. Push come to shove, you may just have to drop a priority for a few days or weeks. Follow what you feel in your heart, for God is present to help you make the Higher Choice and see you through it.

Exploration: Give enough time to each role you take on, and remain flexible.

1. What area of your life seems to suffer the most from interruptions?

2. Could what appears to be an annoying situation be a blessing in disguise? How can remembering your defined priorities help you peacefully handle this circumstance?

126

3. How can you remain true to your purpose through effective time/event management? Is your productivity system performing its job for you?

Faith gives you an inner strength and a sense of balance and perspective in life.
— Gregory Peck

TURNING POINT 4 – ADJUST PRIORITIES

Like it or not, the world evolves,
priorities change and so do you.
– Marilu Henner

Objective: God's purpose for you will take on new dimensions in different seasons of life.

Position: Whereas balancing priorities relates to the near term, priority adjustments are long term, coming with different seasons of life. It is not too difficult to balance how you spend your precious resources to accommodate relatively minor changes in events of normal daily life. However, the emotional and physical stresses associated with major shifts in your personal circumstances require a thorough reassessment. Quite a number of situations may arise to trigger some priority adjustment. Maybe you are a new parent. Perhaps your children are grown and living on their own, enabling you to enjoy more freedom and less responsibility. You may be caring for your elderly parents or other relatives. Or, perhaps a downturn in the economy has reduced your work and income. Life changing experiences are sometimes good and sometimes not so good. Amy Grant's album <u>Behind the Eyes</u>[22] contains more than one song relating to this, like:

Curious Thing

Well, I know that it can be demanding
I know that it can be unkind

I don't really understand it
But Lord sure knows I try
Life is a curious thing
Life, ooh life is a curious thing

Somewhere Down the Road
Why, why, why
Does it go this way
Why, why, why
And all I can say

Somewhere down the road
There'll be answers to the questions
Somewhere down the road
Tho' we cannot see it now
And somewhere down the road
You will find mighty arms reaching for you
And they will hold the answers at the end of the road

A significant adjustment is not always required. The changes made should be germane to the situation, however. Relocating to a new city for a new job may require you to shift both the amount and sequence of time allocated across activities for personal, work, family, and community roles. These adjustments may be temporary or permanent. Seasons come and go, so you will need to adjust priorities more than once. Sometimes we are fortunate to be able to anticipate the life course change, and plan our adjustments in advance. Life is a curious thing! Unexpected things happen, and then we are faced with an adjustment we feel ill equipped to handle. When I began writing this book, I was happily married with three teenagers living at home. Now my children are away at university and I am divorced. I did not see this coming, but I must adjust nonetheless.

Regardless of where you find yourself on this life's journey, God still calls you according to His purposes, and is faithful to show you loving kindness and mercy as you continue to travel on toward your Destination. You never stop being of value! Your mission statement envelopes all your roles. It does not change, because it is a reflection of who you are. Your spiritual gifts have not change, and most of your values probably have not either. Your vision statement should be updated to describe the image of how your purpose will be worked out in your new situation. When I accepted the fact that my life was changing, I went back to the beginning, to A.S.K. God to show me a new vision. The new, beautiful picture sustained me through the adjustment. My role as mother is still important, it just looks a little different than before. I am still coaching and involved in music ministry, but not to the extent I used to be. I did not anticipate working full time again, but it is a special gift from God, providing wealth, challenges, growth, friends, travel, and more writing opportunities.

Since your resource spending is at the heart of your choices, you have to determine how to maximize your time, money, and energy when a change occurs. If you have more to give, then find out what and where. If you feel overwhelmed with basic needs, then direct your resources where they are needed most. The nature of your passion and the types of ministries in which you can be involved will shift in pleasantly surprising ways.

Like balancing priorities, we must look for what God may want to do with the change in circumstances. A few years ago, two faithfully responsive women at my church formed a fantastic women's mentoring ministry. Women of faith need each other for support and encouragement, for teaching, sharing, and fellowship. The wonderfully amazing thing for me to both observe and experience was how God touched each mentor-mentee pair in such a uniquely personal and meaningful way. Among a rich diversity of age, life experience, and spiritual maturity, each woman had something to share, and something to learn. Lasting friendships formed, and lives were changed through this casual and flexible means of encountering God in community. However, none of it would have been possible if the participants had not positioned themselves to give or receive by adjusting their priorities.

I hope that you have been able to Observe and Define your priorities. If life is humming along as it should, just remember that the time for adjustment will come. If you are in a transition now, know that God is right beside you. A.S.K. and He will show you the way.

Exploration: Review your priorities to see if they are consistent with your current life season.

1. Review and update your values list and accompanying clarification statements.

2. Review and update your vision statement.

3. Review and update your goals and Course.

4. Have you had a shift in your roles and/or responsibilities recently? What is God calling you to consider as your new focus?

5. How can you channel some resources differently to help others, and do something meaningful for yourself?

6. In what ways do you need to simply rest in the Lord, and look for the hidden blessings in your current situation?

But seek (aim at and strive after) first of all His kingdom and His righteousness (His way of doing and being right), and then all these things taken together will be given you besides.
– Matthew 6:33 AMP

FITNESS

*Act is the blossom of thought, and joy and suffering
are its fruits; thus does a man garner in the sweet
and bitter fruitage of his own husbandry.*
— James Allen

**Orientation 8 - Choose quality fuel for mind, body,
and soul to maximize your life experiences.**

The link between mind, body, and spirit has been studied for
centuries. We human beings are very complex creatures. You could
spend a lifetime studying every nuance, thus the ideas presented in
this orientation will be simple, based on a few facts and my personal
experience.

The abundant life Christ wants you to experience every day means
sufficient energy, an alert mind, a calm spirit, and confident
productivity. Caring for your body is an area where Higher Choices
are easily identified. A healthy, fit body is both a sign of and a
catalyst for spiritual wellbeing. We live our lives in our minds. That
sounds strange at first, but once you chew on that concept a bit, you
will realize it is true. What we think about ourselves, others, our
job, shapes our perception of our own quality of life. Since we are
constantly thinking, we must control our thoughts, allowing them
to be captive to Christ.

As for energy and vitality, well, how far do you think you will get on
your journey without proper fuel? To enjoy life to the fullest, we need

not only be free of debilitating pain, but we need an energy supply that allows us to achieve our goals and enjoy the adventure.

The four Turning Points you will consider in this orientation are:

1. Physical Fitness - Honor and glorify God by maintaining your wonderful body, and increased life quality is your reward.

2. Mental Fitness - Let God be in your head, guiding your thoughts -- the seeds of everything you create, feel, and experience.

3. Emotional Fitness - You will experience higher feelings and emotions with higher thoughts and actions.

4. Spiritual Fitness - Stay on mission and live your passion to maintain enthusiasm for each day's possibilities.

All four of these aspects of "you" go with you everywhere you go. They are intricately linked to each other, and this connection affects your choices. Children's choir guru, Helen Kemp, said "Mind, body, spirit voice; it takes the whole person to sing and rejoice." Increase your rejoicing through better fitness.

Turning Point 1 – Physical Fitness

*Physical fitness is not only one of the most
important keys to a healthy body, it is the basis
of dynamic and creative intellectual activity.*
– John F. Kennedy

Objective: Honor and glorify God by maintaining your wonderful body, and increased life quality is your reward.

Position: Now that I have experienced life abroad, I can say that Americans are generally more obsessed about their physiques than people elsewhere across the world. Yet at the same time, our nation is increasing in the number of overweight, obese, and sedentary individuals, especially children. Our medical insurance costs are high, because many folks just prefer to take a pill rather than try to properly care for and maintain their physical bodies. It is no secret that when you feel healthy and fit, when you properly care for your body, you are happier, more energetic, and experience a higher quality of life. Whether it is the joy of being able to wear flattering fashions, participate in a walk for charity, or just endure the often-hectic schedule of work and family life, maintaining a healthy fit body has many rewards.

It takes discipline and determination to make Higher Choices regarding physical fitness. It involves many decisions each day. You can dramatically increase your chances of achieving your fitness goals by taking time to plan when you will eat, what you will eat, and when you will exercise. Bill Phillips developed the Body-for-LIFE[40] fitness program. He has written two successful books, co-authored a Body-for-LIFE book for women, and created the EAS' Myoplex line of fitness and sport shakes, snack bars, and supplements. Bill teaches his clients to eat five or six small meals, balancing each with the right portions of good carbohydrates, protein and fats. This principle is consistent with many good healthy eating life style prescriptions. Good health is no secret. You have to eat healthy food and exercise! I love what Bill Phillips said. "You simply cannot escape this reality: Your body is the epicenter of your universe. . . If it is sagging, softening, and aging rapidly, other aspects of your life will soon follow suit." I believe this to be true: how you care for your body indicates how you care for many other aspects of your life.

God gave you your body for you to serve Him and enjoy abundant life. It is wonderfully complex, and able to perform a myriad of tasks. How can you accomplish your goals when your body has run out of fuel? God has called you to a great purpose, so you honor God when your physical body allows you to perform at your best. Being physically fit should not be a burden. Do not go to extremes in either diet or exercise. The key to lasting physical fitness is to create a life style built on the fundamentals. I know you know that already. The math is simple:

Energy Consumed – Energy Used = Energy Stored

Burn more than you consume to lose weight and get into shape. One of the best resources that taught me how to enjoy a wide variety of foods was Portion Savvy[59], by Carrie Latt. It shows you that a wide variety of foods can be enjoyed if you control the amount. Have fun, remember "anything in moderation," and enjoy life more by caring for yourself.

Exploration: Examine and record your eating and exercise habits and see if you want to improve them.

1. Record all food and drink consumption for one week. Note the meal or snack time and portion.

2. Record the time spent engaged in exercise or physical activity. Try a variety of exercise options if you do not already have a set routine that works for you.

3. Analyze your physical fitness log at the end of the week to note the foods and activities you enjoy most and give you energy.

4. Is there a particular time of day that is best for you to exercise? How difficult was it to find time for it?

5. What healthy eating habits can you adopt to increase your fuel supply?

6. Enjoy many good things in moderation! What favorite indulgences can you plan to enjoy with portion control?

If a man achieves victory over this body, who in the world can exercise power over him? He who rules himself rules over the whole world.
— Vinoba Bhave

TURNING POINT 2 – MENTAL FITNESS

*I have strength for all things in Christ who empowers
me [I am ready for anything and equal to anything
through him who infuses inner strength into me].*
– Philippians 4:13, AMP

Objective: Let God be in your head, guiding your thoughts -- the
seeds of everything you create, feel, and experience.

Position: Most of your living is done inside your head, your inner
world. The idea that thoughts are things, that thoughts have a
creative energy that manifests events and circumstances through
the decision-making process, has been written and spoken about
for decades. Well-known psychologists and self-help authors are
consistent in this message – what you expect, believe, and pay
attention to is what you will experience.

I have been interested in the link between one's mind and one's
spiritual fitness for a long time. Through personal experience and
observation, I have come to appreciate the powerful cause and effect
relationship between the two. Books that influenced and inspired me
include The Power of Positive Thinking[39], Battlefield of the Mind[33],
You'll See It When You Believe It[18], Toward a Psychology of Being[1]
and many others. However, what has truly motivated me to focus
on improving my thoughts in order to improve the quality of my life
through Higher Choices is The Bible!

God's Word instructs us how to think as God thinks. The Bible tells us of God's love and God's promises. Bible references describe Psalm 119 as "a devotional on the word of God,⁴⁹" expressing two aspects of God's word: God's directives for life, and God's promises. Verse 30 says, "*The unfolding of your word gives light; it gives understanding to the simple.*" Joshua 1:8 says "*This book of the law shall not depart out of your mouth, but you shall meditate on it day and night, that you may be careful to do according to all that is written in it; for then you shall make your way prosperous, and then you shall have good success.*"

Self improvement and business success gurus tell you to use positive affirmations to motivate yourself to take action consistent with your desires. It can be as simple as Brian Tracy's suggestion to say, "I feel terrific!" or Louis Hay's "I love and approve of myself." I have discovered, however, that affirmations based upon God's Word are more than just feel good statements. Scriptural affirmations give light, and re-enforce right living. Reminding myself of God's promises aligns my mood and attitude with True North. Scriptural affirmations also remind me how God expects me to behave in my interactions with others. Consider any of the following Bible verses:

Deuteronomy 31:8 – "*The LORD himself goes before you and will be with you; he will never leave you nor forsake you. Do not be afraid; do not be discouraged.*"

Psalm 23 – "*The LORD is my shepherd, I lack nothing. He makes me lie down in green pastures, he leads me beside quiet waters, he refreshes my soul. He guides me along the right paths for his name's sake. Even though I walk through the darkest valley, I will fear no evil, for you are with me; your rod and your staff, they comfort me. You prepare a table before me in the presence of my enemies. You anoint my head with oil; my cup overflows. Surely your goodness and love will follow me all the days of my life, and I will dwell in the house of the LORD forever.*"

Isaiah 43:18-19 – *"Forget the former things; do not dwell on the past. See, I am doing a new thing! Now it springs up; do you not perceive it? I am making a way in the wilderness and streams in the wasteland."*

Proverbs 3:27 – *"Do not withhold good from those to whom it is due, when it is in your power to act."*

Matthew 11:28-30 – *"Come to me, all you who are weary and burdened, and I will give you rest. Take my yoke upon you and learn from me, for I am gentle and humble in heart, and you will find rest for your souls. For my yoke is easy and my burden is light."*

John 6:35 – *"Then Jesus declared, "I am the bread of life. Whoever comes to me will never go hungry, and whoever believes in me will never be thirsty."*

Philippians 4:4-7 – *"Rejoice in the Lord always. I will say it again: Rejoice! Let your gentleness be evident to all. The Lord is near. Do not be anxious about anything, but in every situation, by prayer and petition, with thanksgiving, present your requests to God. And the peace of God, which transcends all understanding, will guard your hearts and your minds in Christ Jesus."*

James 5:15-16 – *"And the prayer offered in faith will make the sick person well; the Lord will raise them up. If they have sinned, they will be forgiven. Therefore confess your sins to each other and pray for each other so that you may be healed. The prayer of a righteous person is powerful and effective."*

Think positively about yourself and others, and banish negative thoughts as soon as you recognize them. Focus on your vision, keeping it foremost in your mind. I do not recall who is famous for saying "It's all in your head," but they're right!

Exploration: Renew your mind each day with Scriptural affirmations. Expect good things.

1. Observe and record your thoughts a few times each day for one week to increase awareness of the thoughts you allow. Consider writing out an affirmation or scripture verse to trigger positive thoughts.

2. What do you observe about your thoughts about others and yourself?

3. Be creative in selecting your own affirmations. How can listening to inspirational music or audio books help?

Men imagine that thought can be kept secret,
but it cannot; it rapidly crystallizes into habit,
and habit solidifies into circumstance.
— James Allen

Turning Point 3 – Emotional Fitness

"Where love is," said Tolstoy, "God is," and, we might add, where God and love are, there is happiness. So a practical principle in creating happiness is to practice love.
– Norman Vincent Peale

Objective: You will experience higher feelings and emotions with higher thoughts and actions.

Position: "An emotion is a mental and physiological state associated with a wide variety of feelings, thoughts, and behaviors. It is a prime determinant of the sense of subjective well-being and appears to play a central role in many human activities. . . There is much controversy concerning how emotions are defined and classified.[45]" The word 'emotion' is derived from the French word meaning 'out' and 'move.' Emotions effect physiological changes in preparation for action. Thus, the emotions you allow and choose direct your behavior and actions.

Many of our emotional responses are automatic simply due to years of learning, through culture and education, what are appropriate or inappropriate responses to every kind of stimuli. Although our emotional responses may be automatic, we can control their form of expression, and how long they last. You can retrain yourself to choose either the emotion itself, or the magnitude and length of the response. It is difficult to separate or isolate thoughts, emotions, and spirit, because their interaction is so involved. However, it is true

141

that better thoughts will lead to better emotions. The emotions you allow yourself to experience will determine the quality of your spirit, i.e., how motivated, energized and full of life you are at any given time. A healthy spirit supports inspired, positive thoughts. Picture the three as rings, or gimbals, of a gyroscope and you can see how the interaction of thoughts, emotions, and spirit can determine your orientation.

Controlling your emotions does not mean you are insensitive. We all know that many emotional responses are desirable to others and ourselves. They are what make us truly human. We communicate more deeply through emotions and feelings. Jesus was emotional. He was passionate about the thieves in the temple (John 2:14-16), and full of sorrow at Gethsemane (Matthew 26:36-39). The message of this Turning Point is to make you aware that you can have power over your emotions in order to make Higher Choices. Be mindful of your feelings, so you can choose whether or not to change your emotional state at any given time. Changing them as you are able allows you to maximize happiness and minimize despair; to relinquish fear and embrace love.

I grew up watching television in the 1970s. No surprise then that I was, and still am, a Star Trek fan. What young girl could resist the appeal of a then vibrant and handsome William Shatner? The Star Trek character Spock constantly struggled with his inner conflict of being half-Vulcan, part of a culture in which emotional expression is frowned upon, and being half-Human, part of a culture in which emotional expression is encouraged. I believe Spock controlled his emotions, because it enabled him to think, make wise decisions, work productively, and perform at his highest capacity. At the same time, he acknowledged the benefits of allowing himself to display the right emotion in the right situation. Like Spock, we tend to get into trouble when we fail to acknowledge a negative feeling, and simply try to ignore it or cover it up. No one is helped by ignoring or suppressing emotions. We must first acknowledge what we feel, consider the cause, and then decide to stay in that state or alter it. Easier said than done, of course! Making a choice about anything means that you have identified your options - you are aware of both option A and option B. You have the opportunity to select one or the other. Selecting the better emotion, the Higher Choice, begins before the emotion is manifest by selecting better thoughts. Yet, once they are real, paying attention to your emotional state allows you to remain in control. More positive emotions are within grasp when you simply become aware of what triggers various emotional responses in you, and decide whether or not each "state" is a Higher Choice.

Exploration: Observe and record your emotions, and see how often you can choose the state you experience.

1. Observe and record your emotions a few times each day for one week to increase awareness of your feelings.

2. What positive emotions are you noticing this week? What were you thinking at the time?

3. What negative emotions are you noticing this week? How was your energy level affected?

4. Are there some feelings you now wish to minimize or maximize? What will have to change?

Anger, resentment, and guilt make you sick, modern physicians tell us, which proves once again that the most up-to-date book on personal well-being is the Holy Bible.
— Norman Vincent Peale

TURNING POINT 4 – SPIRITUAL FITNESS

Attitude is everything.
– Diane von Furstenberg

Passion is energy. Feel the power that comes
from focusing on what excites you.
– Oprah Winfrey

Objective: Stay on mission and live your passion to maintain enthusiasm for each day's possibilities.

Position: Spiritual Fitness is not spirituality (the quality or fact of being spiritual). When people say, "she is in good spirits," they are referring to a woman's attitude or outlook, her energy level and motivation perhaps. Key synonyms are attitude, energy, life force, will, and motivation. Your spiritual fitness is good when you go about your day with a good measure of enthusiasm and power, with anticipation and positive expectation.

Christopher Reeves, the accomplished movie actor best known for his role as Superman, was an awesome example of a man whose spirit was often "fit," despite his personal tragedy. In 1995, he became a quadriplegic after being thrown by his horse in a dressage competition. Reeves suffered inner anguish in the early days of recovery, unable to move or breathe on his own. Yet Reeves was able to overcome and energize his spirit as he saw progress with his therapy, and possibilities for a medical breakthrough. He and his wife worked tirelessly to establish a foundation to further spinal cord injury research. The key to his positive and motivating attitude was that he chose to see the possibilities. Taking action to follow his newfound passion fueled his motivation as well.

Wouldn't you love to wake up every morning pumped and ready to start the day? You can, by acting on two principles: fit instruments perform better, and passion boosts energy. The connection between the four fitness areas mentioned here is inescapable. Diminished health in one will degrade the health of another. You experience quality of life through higher qualities of physical, mental, emotional, and spiritual fitness. As for passion, knowing your Destination gives you a vital sense of purpose and passion that fuels your spirit. Taking action to fulfill your dreams and God's will for your life is a natural motivator. Working in your gifted areas brings joy. Knowing that you are contributing the world in your own special way is rewarding. Abundant life is more a matter of attitude than circumstance.

Life is too short to waste a single day in poor spirits when it is within your control not to. Improving any area of fitness and wellbeing is challenging. The good news is that there are gifted people who's passion is to help you. Seek them out. We all face tough times and have "things" to work through, so there will be lousy days. We do not control all our circumstances, but we do choose how we respond to them. Like Christopher Reeves, you can choose the way you look at your situation, and what you decide to do about it. The winningest female college basketball coach for the University of Tennessee, Pat Summit, was recently diagnosed with early onset of dementia. In a television interview, her son said that he felt her future was still bright, because he remembered what his mother always told him; "It is what it is, but it will be what you make it." Let Higher Choices in your physical, mental, and emotional fitness help you "make it" what you will, and give you the life force that brings abundance in all your experiences.

Exploration: Pay attention to your energy and motivational levels in all areas of your life.

1. Observe and record your spirit level a few times each day for one week to increase awareness of the life force you promote.

2. On a scale from 1-10, how high is your daily energy level?

3. What is your motivation and determination like this week? What is the cause?

4. How are your thoughts and emotions influencing your spirit?

You have made known to me the path of life;
you will fill me with joy in your presence, with
eternal pleasures at your right hand.
– Psalm 16: 11

PROGRESS

The expectations of life depend upon diligence; the mechanic
that would perfect his work must first sharpen his tools.
– Confucius

Orientation 9 - Making progress towards your
Destination comes through diligence and flexibility.
Personal fitness coach and author, Steve Ilg, reminds his readers that
life is a journey when he writes, "you have your whole life to become
wholistically fit.[28]" He says this, because he wants his clients to do
what they can on a consistent basis, paying attention to how they
are changing and improving a little at a time each day. Aim to enjoy
the process and small accomplishments.

I almost named this month's orientation "growth" to represent the
process of maturing in faith and personal development. From a
human perspective, accomplishment and self-actualization lead to
success. From a 'kingdom' perspective, becoming a new creation and
increasing in personal holiness lead to perfection. John Wesley said,
*"And as, in the natural birth, a man is born at once and then grows
larger and stronger by degrees, so in the spiritual birth, a man is born
at once and then gradually increases in spiritual stature and strength.
The new birth, therefore, is the first point of sanctification, which may
increase 'more and more unto the perfect day[38]" (Prov. 4:18).* While we
are in this world, both are important.

Personal growth, however, is only half the message of progress. The other half is acknowledging and experiencing the freedom that comes from collaborating with the Holy Spirit. Progress is a subjective term – a matter of judgment. Who defines whether you are making progress? The Higher Choices concept of progress is that you are to do what you know you should be doing to expand and improve, while exercising faith that "*in all things God works for the good of those who love him, who are called according to his purpose*" (Romans 8:28).

The four Turning Points you will consider in this orientation are:

1. Spiritual Formation - Achieve true progress as each Higher Choice makes you more Christ-like.

2. Skills Development - Be a continuous learner, and experience fulfillment by investing in personal growth.

3. Perfect Results - Perform well your role, as unto the Lord, and the outcome will be just what it should.

4. Perfect Timing - Wait patiently for the Lord to accomplish all good things at the perfect time.

Growth means change, and that is not easy. Progress takes constant and earnest effort. The good news is that when you persist in faith, you can rest in the assurance that God is faithful to his promises.

TURNING POINT 1 – SPIRITUAL FORMATION

Spiritual formation for the Christian basically refers to the Spirit-driven process of forming the inner world of the human self in such a way that it becomes like the inner being of Christ himself.
– Dallas Willard

Objective: Achieve true progress as each Higher Choice makes you more Christ-like.

Position: You know that thoughts determine actions, repeated actions turn into habits, and habits become character. Making progress toward your Destination, by definition, calls you to be continuously growing into the person God intends, operating at full God-capacity. The Bible teaches that our number one purpose in this world is to learn to fully love God and our fellow man. I believe that all of the events and relationships we experience are potential teachers, allowed or sent by God to shape and mold our character. Thus, as we obediently do God's will, we are changing and growing; we are transformed.

A person who continues to grow in her faith and discipleship exhibits that change in her character and behavior. Making progress requires intention, however. If you want to grow in Spirit, you must work at it. On my first day as a new summer hand with an oil company years ago, the foreman introduced me to an older man who had been working this particular field for 30 years. Being duly impressed I said, "Wow, 30 years of experienced!" To which the foreman replied, "No, Herman has one year of experience 30 times." Herman was not interested in growing his career. That is okay. Hopefully he was interested in becoming the best human being he could.

Transformed people exhibit the Fruits of the Spirit. As you recall, the fourth Turning Point in the A.S.K. Orientation is Abiding. Abiding is living out God's truth for you through the grace and power of the Holy Spirit. He is the vine; we are the branches. You will experience an *"inward change from all unholy to holy tempers: from pride to humility, from passionateness to meekness, from peevishness and discontent to patience and resignation; in a word, from an earthly, sensual, devilish mind to the mind that was in Christ Jesus* [Phil. 2:5],[37]" as Wesley states. Dr. Wayne Dyer helps us visualize this concept by explaining the origin of the word transform. In his book, You'll See it When You Believe It[18], he says that 'trans' mean beyond, thus to be transformed simply means to go beyond one's form, one's humanness.

What can you do to allow and promote the work of the Spirit within you? Practice spiritual disciplines. I recommend the classic reference by Richard J. Foster, Celebration of Discipline: The Path to Spiritual Growth[20]. This wonderful resource will teach you what the disciplines are, why they are important, and how to practice them. Outward progress toward your Destination is important, but inward progress is the real goal. You will surely increase your capacity and make God known by your fruit.

Exploration: Examine your inner progress. Research spiritual disciplines and adopt one or two.

1. Select one or two of Foster's Inward Disciplines to try throughout the next 30 days - Meditation, Prayer, Fasting, and Study.

2. Expect promptings from the Holy Spirit. Be open and follow through. Record your insights and experiences in a journal.

3. What image does "Christ-like character" bring to your mind? Describe your vision so you can begin to move toward that.

4. Spiritual growth is Spirit-driven. How are you letting the Holy Spirit nourish you?

The Christian life is always "life in the Spirit" (Gal 5:25), in all its variety and unpredictability.
– Arthur Holder

TURNING POINT 2 – SKILLS DEVELOPMENT

A winner is someone who recognizes his God-given
talents, works his tail off to develop them into skills,
and uses these skills to accomplish his goals.
– Larry Bird

Objective: Be a continuous learner, and experience fulfillment by investing in personal growth.

Position: When my business coaching partner and I worked to define and clarify our work values, we selected "growth" as one of the top five. Our value clarification statement was, "you are either growing or you are behind." In this fast-paced information age, sticking only with what you know is not good enough. Successful people are intentional about continuous learning.

All of us enjoy having a skill we can perform well and continue to improve upon. It is particularly exciting to realize that you are evolving and expanding skills in your area of purpose and passion. Although God does not expect perfection, you have a responsibility to use your spiritual gifts, and use them well. A perceived lack of skill is not an excuse not to serve. In my workshops I often share Charles Stanley's teaching, The Blessings of Our Inadequacy[53], to encourage people to start with what they have. Acknowledging our deficiencies causes us to rely upon the power of the Holy Spirit, and removes limitations we place on doing God's work. You know that many biblical figures, such as Moses and Jeremiah, did not feel equipped to serve the Lord as instructed. God often calls men and women thought to be the least likely persons to accomplish the task. Christ makes us sufficient to perform, and in so doing, God gets the glory. Nevertheless, we should continually expand our capability and strive for excellence in whatever endeavor we undertake.

There are a few reasons why skills development is particularly important to Higher Choices:

- Mission is about process, so the work invested to learn and improve your talents keeps you on mission. If your "thing" is finance, then you are living on purpose when you attend an accounting class or read relevant books and articles.

- Attending seminars or conferences allows you to connect with others in your gift area. You get to share ideas and consider new avenues of expression.

- Growing and advancing are natural results of well-defined goals, thus working towards your goals is skills development. Selecting a challenging piano piece to learn in six month's time, and then following through with consistent practice, will naturally increase your piano performance. The goal of writing this book caused me to improve my writing skills. I went to my bookshelves and pulled out the classic references on writing I already owned. I bought a new book on how to write magazine articles for publication, and I have frequently picked up issues of writers' magazines. I had to improve my skills to reach the goal.

- The desire to improve your skills is an avenue to self-discovery, which in itself leads to self-motivation. You learn what you are capable of, your confidence increases, and you are ready for the next challenge.

Matthew 25:29 says, *"For everyone who has will be given more, and he will have an abundance."* We should all be investing in personal growth, for it is a source of joy and keeps our enthusiasm high. A little confidence in your abilities gives you a sense of boldness to step out and do the work to which you are called.

Exploration: Make a plan to enhance and improve your gifts, skills, and talents.

1. You have already identified your spiritual gifts. List other natural talents and skills you enjoy.

2. Review the goals in your Course to ensure they include your most important skills. Design them to pull you beyond your current abilities.

3. If you are having trouble identifying an area for skills development, ask your friends and loved ones what skills they see in you. Is there a class or workshop you can take?

4. What latent talents can you enjoy again? Figure out where to begin again.

> Intellectual growth should commence at birth
> and cease only at death.
> — Albert Einstein

Turning Point 3 – Perfect Results

*We must not, in trying to think about how we
can make a big difference, ignore the small daily
differences we can make which, over time, add up
to big differences that we often cannot foresee.*
– Marian Wright Edelman

Objective: Perform well your role, as unto the Lord, and the outcome
will be just what it should.

Position: One thing I love about God is the seemingly bizarre ideas
and plans He calls people to go along with. His ways truly are not
our ways! This is a liberating concept to me, because it means if
I am faithful to the Course, God promises to be responsible for
the outcome. Charles Stanley says, "Obey God and leave all the
consequences to him." We play a small role in God's plan. Therefore,
we are not in a position to question our path, but responsible for
staying on it.

The story of Gideon is a wonderful example of how God's ways can
be contrary to common sense. The seventh chapter of the book of
Judges tells the story. *"God said to Gideon, 'You have too large an army
with you. I can't turn Midian over to them like this—they'll take all the
credit, saying, 'I did it all myself,' and forget about me. Make a public
announcement: 'Anyone afraid, anyone who has any qualms at all, may
leave Mount Gilead now and go home.'" Twenty-two companies headed
for home. Ten companies were left. God said to Gideon: 'There are still*

too many. Take them down to the stream and I'll make a final cut."
After God had Gideon reduce his army from 32,000 to just 300,
their only 'weapons' were trumpets and empty jars with torches. "*The
whole Midianite camp jumped to its feet. They yelled and fled. When
the three hundred blew the trumpets, God aimed each Midianite's sword
against his companion, all over the camp. They ran for their lives…*"
(The Message, 7:2-4, 21-22). The perfect result was achieved in quite
an unusual way!

Your commitment to follow God in humility allows others to see
God's handiwork, allows God to be glorified. You never know who
is watching you, or how you and your actions may affect another.
Often when I thought something I did was a disastrous flop, it
turned out to inspire someone I never considered. The challenge for
you and me is to trust and let go. Faith in God and, God's larger
plan, is liberating. When you do not have to worry about the results,
you are free to enjoy the process. You can release all fear and doubt,
and simply let your light shine.

Many times you will not be aware that you are making progress,
because you are separated from the result in either time or space.
Genesis 39 tells of Joseph's success. His jealous brothers dumped
him on the side of the road, and left him to die. A caravan of
Ishmaelites carried him to Egypt, where he was bought as a slave to
Potiphar. Although Joseph became a servant in a foreign land and was
wrongly accused and thrown into prison, he accepted his position.
He remained righteous, performed his duties with excellence, and
as result, Potiphar and Pharoah could see God through Joseph.
"*Then his master saw that the Lord was with him and that the Lord
gave him success in everything he did, Joseph found favor in his eyes.*"
(39:3). No doubt, Joseph had a different plan for his life, but with
benefit of hindsight and the whole story, we see the perfection of it.
The nation of Israel was saved from starvation, and Joseph united
with his family. I had a different plan for this season of my life as

well. I tried desperately to save my marriage. Not only did I pray for God to facilitate reconciliation, but many dear friends prayed on our behalf as well. My desire was consistent with God's Word and His intention that two shall become (and remain) as one. Yet, as I yield to the Father's wisdom and follow my new path, I already experience a portion of the perfection of it. I trust God to be faithful to His promises.

Exploration: Trust God's plan to yield perfect results.

1.   Is there a project or task you are hesitant to start? How can trusting God get you moving?

2.   Is doubt or fear holding you back from a decision your gut tells you is right? What desired outcome do you need to let go of and let God handle?

3.   What would you dare to do if you knew the results would be perfect?

> *Blessed is she who has believed that what the
> Lord has said to her will be accomplished.*
> – Luke 1:45

Turning Point 4 – Perfect Timing

*For the vision is yet for an appointed time and it hastens
to the end [fulfillment]; it will not deceive or disappoint.
Though it tarry, wait [earnestly] for it, because it will surely
come; it will not be behindhand or its appointed day.*
– Habakkuk 2:3 AMP

Objective: Wait patiently for the Lord to accomplish all good things at the perfect time.

Position: The idea for creating a faith-based calendar and agenda came to me in 2004. I did not produce a workable prototype until the end of 2009. Client feedback and my own analysis of the 2010 Higher Choices Compass revealed the need for reformatting and expanding the concepts. Only now, eight years after the initial idea, has it finally taken shape. Of course, the excitement I felt in the beginning, along with the great knowledge I thought I possessed (ha!), convinced me that this project would take only one or two years. My vision was correct, but the timing has been in God's hands.

I served as a project manager for most of my corporate career. Part of my job was to visualize the range of tasks required to meet the project's objectives, and arrange them in time and relation to one another. Tasks can be performed both in sequence and in parallel. Every project has what is known as the Critical Path, made up of the string of dependent tasks with the longest durations. Although other work is being carried out simultaneously, the project cannot be completed any sooner than the time required to complete tasks on the Critical Path. Thinking of God's plan for my life as a multi-task project helps me understand that my responsibility is limited to a certain set of activities. The items for which I am solely responsible may or may not be on the Critical Path.

Although the shortest distance between two points is a straight line, it is unlikely that is what God has in mind. You cannot anticipate the people and events you will encounter on your adventure. The personal connections you make will cause your Course to take on new directions. The scope of work may increase, or need to be modified in some way. There could be a gap in activity while you wait for the completion of some event.

Co-creating with God means keeping pace with God's plan - whatever that is! Someone said that God is never late. I trust that is true, because I have faith that God is loving and wise, thus He will direct me to my highest good. Many scripture verses tell us to wait upon the Lord. We can get ourselves into trouble when we try to make things happen too quickly, out of God's timing. Just look at what happened to Sarah, Abraham, and Hagar (named Sarai and Abram in these passages). In Genesis Chapter 12, God calls Abraham saying "*I will make you into a great nation and I will bless you; (v2)*" and "*To your offspring I will give this land.*" We read more of God's promise in Chapter 13: "*I will make your offspring like the dust of the earth, so that if anyone could count the dust, then your offspring could be counted.*" Abraham was 75 years old when first called by God. After waiting 10 years, and seeing no evidence of God's promise, Sarah decided to take matters into her own hand.

"*Now Sari, Abram's wife, had borne him no children. But she had an Egyptian maidservant named Hagar; so she said to Abram, 'The Lord has kept me from having children. Go sleep with my maidservant; perhaps I can build a family through her.' Abram agreed to what Sarai said. So after Abram had been living in Canaan ten years, Sarai his wife took her Egyptian maidservant Hagar and gave her to her husband to be his wife. He slept with Hagar, and she conceived. When she knew she was pregnant, she began to despise her mistress. Then Sarai said the Abram, 'You are responsible for the wrong I am suffering, I put my servant in your arms, and now that she knows she is pregnant, she despises me. May the Lord judge between you and me.'"* (Genesis 16: 1-5).

Sarah did become pregnant and bear a son when Abraham was 100 years old! Twenty-five years from his initial calling from God, and fifteen years from the time Ishmael was born. Now, the Bible does not indicate that the time delay was precipitated by the couple's impatient course of action, it just was not the timing they expected or desired. It is clear that they did indeed receive God's perfect results - their precious son Isaac, and promised nation to follow. Waiting is hard! We do not like it, especially in this world of instant gratification. It is doubly hard when you are passionate about your mission and want to make a difference. Stay on Course, no matter where it leads, and you will reach your Destination in perfect timing.

Exploration: Consider how the progress of past or current goals may be right on schedule.

1. Some say hindsight is 20-20. Can you identify any past endeavors that completed at a different time than you expected?

2. How has the timing of a goal or dream caused it to produce a different, yet surprisingly good result?

3. Often waiting on God is for our own good, so we can rest and not fret. Is there some task you are striving to complete now that perhaps you need a break from instead?

Wait and hope for and expect the Lord; be brave and of good courage and let your heart be stout and enduring. Yes, wait for and hope for and expect the Lord.
– Psalm 27:14

NAVIGATION

Problems do not go away. They must be worked
through or else they remain, forever a barrier to
the growth and development of the spirit.
– M. Scott Peck

Orientation 10 - Maintain your Course through information acquisition and analysis.

Navigation is part of any journey. It does not matter if it is trying to get to a new restaurant in an unfamiliar part of town, or piloting a jet airplane from Houston to LA. Once you have begun to travel, you must check to see if your heading is consistent with the plan. You need to keep your eyes open and read the signs to know where you are. Our lives move forward, sometimes at break-neck speed. Periodically pausing to observe and reorient lets you maintain a measure of control over your direction. Growing in faith and discipleship takes dedication and focus. Even with discipline, life's activities, pressures, pleasures, and concerns easily distract us. Choices conflicting with your priorities will take you off target. All of the sudden it seems you lose your bearing, wander away from your objective, and then must work to get back on track. It happens to all of us. We get lost and need to find our way home.

The four Turning Points you will consider in this orientation are:

1. Awareness - Know intimately the road you have been traveling to determine if you are still on Course.

2. Obstacles - Overcome obstacles through faith and discernment, knowing God will help you persevere.

3. Re-Orienting - No matter what has taken you off Course, new beginnings are always available.

4. God's Leading - Your life is abundant and adventurous when you anticipate God's activity in and around you, and you decide to join in.

Remember that 'Life is an Adventure,' and the path is never straight. Increasing your awareness of choices in real time and identifying real obstacles provide the information you need to keep from veering from your Course. Journaling is an excellent navigation aid. Keeping a journal and reviewing it frequently will show whether or not you are being true to your purpose. Knowing what you actually did this week will guide you to next week's Higher Choices. Commit the little bit of time and attention required to make your journey a successful and rewarding one.

Our personal choices are not the only ones that divert us. We are also affected by our loved one's decisions. What our employer decides to do, and countless outside events can rock our worlds. Your job is to recognize when you are veering off track or rendered immobile by an obstacle. Ask yourself what went wrong, or what is holding you back. Maybe it is something within your control to change. Perhaps it is not, and you must decide how this new situation fits in with your priorities. Higher Choices demand life navigation skills. You are not alone, however!

Turning Point 1 – Awareness

Let us not look back in anger or forward in fear,
but around in awareness.
– James Thurbur

Objective: Know intimately the road you have been traveling to determine if you are still on Course.

Position: Pondering how essential awareness is for proper navigation makes me think of a submarine deep beneath the sea, maneuvering through the dark, often cavernous ocean depths. The pilot and navigator rely on a panel of sophisticated instruments to supply data they must constantly interpret to calculate the submarine's location and trajectory. The captain and crew cannot complete their mission without a keen awareness of not only the ship's position, but also the oceanic environment through which they must travel.

Good life navigation skills require that you practice awareness. You must be aware of your position relative to your Destination to know if you are still on Course. Noticing each day's thoughts, feelings, and actions will expose the environment you are creating for yourself. Then, you can decide if it is working for you, or consider making a few adjustments. Journaling is a very useful discipline for anyone desiring to grow closer to God, and grow in God's likeness. Recording how you spend your time reveals more than where the time went. It will show your true priorities across all roles and life areas. Keeping a personal journal to record ideas, insights, prayers, and the like will also increase your sense of mental, emotional, and spiritual fitness. Practicing mindfulness, the intentional observation of your thoughts and surroundings throughout the day, is useful and noble. I benefit greatly from this practice. However, taking a few moments each day to write down what you are doing, thinking, and feeling, equips you with valuable, hard facts upon which to base your next Higher Choices.

Take advantage of the myriad of cell phone apps, online journals, and "the cloud." The productivity system you designed earlier can most likely handle both plan and actual data. A printed weekly calendar is the perfect place to record how you spend your time. Notes or To-Do apps may be good tools for recording your actions and noteworthy discoveries. Use a fitness log to remain aware of how you are caring for yourself, and how you are benefiting from that. Use blank pages or a special prayer journal to guide your conversations with God, noting persons brought to mind for which you can intercede, and recording those flashes of insight God reveals to you in such interesting and creative ways.

Successful people stay on track. Speaker and author Jim Rohn published a short article entitled, "Keeping a Journal: One of the Three Treasures to Leave Behind[41]." The first two treasures are your pictures (capturing memories) and your library (the books that instructed you and helped you define your ideas). Then, Jim writes, "The third treasure is your journals: the ideas that you picked up, the information that you meticulously gathered. But of the three, journal writing is one of the greatest indications that you're a serious student. Taking pictures, that is pretty easy. Buying a book at a book store, that's pretty easy. It is a little more challenging to be a student of your own life, your own future, your own destiny. Take the time to keep notes and to keep a journal. You'll be so glad you did. What a treasure to leave behind when you go. What a treasure to enjoy today!"

Practicing awareness, especially in the form of journaling, is the first step in navigation. It may seem that all of this writing is going to take too much time. You are busy already, right? Thirty minutes a day is all you need. Much of it can be done as you go about your day, although, setting aside a few minutes at day's end is a rewarding practice. Do not trust your memory! Our minds are not as reliable as we think – especially as we get older. Keep an open mind and try journaling for 30 days. You will be surprised by what you notice.

Exploration: Journal everyday to heighten awareness, equipping yourself to stay on Course.

1. In the Observe Priorities Turning Point, you took a broad-stroke snapshot of time as a resource. Continue the practice of recording where your hours go to increase awareness of time and priorities. Use an agenda with a 'notes' or 'appointments' section, a journal, or phone. Be creative and select something that is convenient and easy.

2. Use a fitness log to record your exercise and eating choices. Add to that a space for recording your thoughts, emotions, and spiritual outlook.

3. Record ideas and insights you come across at work. Take notes from inspiring articles. Jot down 'To Dos' as they come to you, regardless of when you think you might actually get to it.

4. Keep a prayer journal to record your spiritual journey, and see how God is moving in around you.

5. Your journal is only for you to see. Are you hesitant to record anything, and if so, why?

6. What observances can you make about the Course you are traveling, as revealed by real information?

7. How is writing your prayers increasing your faith connection?

I think self-awareness is probably the most important thing towards being a champion.
– Billie Jean King

TURNING POINT 2 – OBSTACLES

*Consider it pure joy, my brothers, whenever you face trials of
many kinds, because you know that the testing of your faith
develops perseverance. Perseverance must finish its work so
that you may be mature and complete, not lacking anything.*
– James 1:2-3

Objective: Overcome obstacles through faith and discernment,
knowing God will help you persevere.

Position: I remember playing a fun game when I was in Kindergarten,
called, "Let's go on a bear hunt." Sitting cross-legged and marching
left and right palms on our knees, we followed the teacher through
an imaginary obstacle course of trees, rocks, rivers and such. Each
time we encountered an obstruction on our bear hunt, we echoed
her phrase of wholeheartedness to help us move beyond it: "I see a
tree--a great big tree. We can't go around it. We can't go under it.
We can't go over it. I guess we'll have to climb it."

An obstacle is something that is in your way, something that presents
a challenge, and the potential for derailment. You will encounter
obstacles of all shapes and sizes throughout your life journey.
Different from ordinary distractions however, the obstacles you
face when you are on Course, being intentional about living your
mission, can be subtle. It seems that being proactive, co-creating
your life with God, can move your sprint track into the hurdle lane.
Your challenge in overcoming these obstacles is three-fold:

- Differentiating between obstacles and excuses,

- Understanding the true nature of the obstacle,

- Knowing where to turn for guidance and strength.

You have to analyze the roadblock to understand its source and form before you can determine the best way to deal with it. Then you have to know how to go about either removing the obstacle, or creatively plowing through. Will it be worth the cost necessary to remove it? Some obstacles go away if you ignore them. Often we create our own roadblocks by making hasty choices. Remember Sarah's and Abraham's predicament when they tried to rush God's timing? Additionally, we can have conflicting values that are creating impediments and not realize it. For example, you may value quality time with your spouse, but your boss in the marketing department has you spending the majority of your evenings with clients. The boss gets your attention, while your spouse waits.

Procrastination and fear are major obstacles, especially when you want to grow in an area that takes you out of your comfort zones. It is amazing what excuses we can conjure to cover the real reason we are stalling. Procrastination is a defense against doing the tough, unpleasant job. It is so much more comfortable to start with the easy job, and leave the hard for the end! And nothing will stop you dead in your tracks like fear. Like a big black bear that suddenly emerges from the forest, fear of success, fear of failure, fear of what others may think all get your heart pounding and your feet moving in the opposite direction. These are not real obstacles. You have allowed your mind to dwell on all of the "what if" scenarios with potential negative outcomes, rather than embracing the strength and power the Holy Spirit gives you in the present moment.

Obstacles are not always negative. God allows temptations and trials to mold and shape us. The Bible consistently testifies that we are to persevere in doing God's will. James 1:12 tells us, *"God blesses those who patiently endure testing and temptation. Afterward they will receive the crown of life that God has promised to those who love him."* You will stay on Course to the degree you are effective in removing and overcoming obstacles. How will you do it? Pray about your obstacle. Use your practice of awareness to discern true obstacles from excuses. Remember the Knock part of the A.S.K. process. Find out how you are to grow through the experience. Look for a turning point of opportunity. Trust God to not only reveal the truth, but to assist and sustain you as you follow the guidance you sense He is giving. Persevere in your quest, abiding in the Lord, and He will prove that what seems to be an encumbrance is an open doorway to a golden highway.

Exploration: Identify true and false obstacles, and work with God to overcome them.

1. What percentage of time are you living on mission? What obstacle may be hindering your progress?

2. Is the main challenge you face right now real or imagined? What is its true nature and source?

3. Are you going through a particularly trying time? Recognize the reality of the situation, ask God for strength, discernment, and peace. Know that a different kind of progress is being made, and that you will overcome.

Obstacles are like wild animals. They are cowards but they will bluff you if they can. If they see you are afraid of them... they are liable to spring upon you; but if you look them squarely in the eye, they will slink out of sight.
– Orison Swett Marden

Turning Point 3 – Reorienting

It takes a little time sometimes to get your
feet back on the ground. It takes a little time
sometimes to turn the Titanic back around. . .
Give it, give it time.
— Amy Grant

Objective: No matter what has taken you off Course, new beginnings are always available.

Position: It is never too late to change your heading and get back on Course. The task may be small or large, depending upon how far you have wandered. Course corrections are easier to make when you catch them early. Getting derailed is one thing, but continuing to travel an errant detour, whether due to deception, disobedience, or something completely outside of your control, is your choice.

Discovering that we are in unfavorable territory catches us unawares, because the journey progresses slowly, one step at a time. A former software development colleague wonderfully pointed out that a major group project that was in trouble at the time "didn't become a million dollars over budget over night!" They failed to keep a close eye on costs that were eroding the fixed priced contract profit, one day, one week, and one month at a time. They allowed themselves to be deceived about their capabilities, and disobedient to corporate management procedures. Upper management swooped in and helped them correct their course, knowing there was value in continuing with the client. There is great value in you getting back on Course as well.

Thank the Lord above that His mercies are new every morning! Our God is the God of second chances. When you veer off Course, your Higher Choice is to acknowledge it, and reorient to True North.

- Assess your position by reviewing your weekly time logs and journals. Note what was good and what you might like to change. Set your objectives for the next week accordingly.

- Focus on the Seek part of the A.S.K. process to see if current practices are fruitful. Your initial idea may have been great, but a few adjustments may be required.

- Check your spirit and sense of peace as a barometer of Higher Choices. Your heart knows when you are honoring your own personal values and doing the best you can at any given time, in any given situation.

My Sunday evening commitment to a review and plan process has been extremely valuable. Scanning my planner and journal, I am often amazed at how prayers were answered, important plans went off without a hitch, and surprising moments brightened my week. Taking lead from Dale Carnegie, I evaluate the past week by asking myself, "What was great about my performance," and "What could be improved?" Based upon my assessment, I briefly prioritize just three goals for the coming week. Adopt this practice. The 30 minutes or so you spend each week will keep you from drifting too far off course. As you look back, you will be amazed at the wonderful things you have accomplished, and the changes you are realizing. Note what you would like to improve, but more importantly, focus on the positive, looking forward to the next week with fresh motivation and commitment fueled by your accomplishments.

Do not be hard on yourself. Rabbi Karyn D. Kedar has written a lovely book entitled, <u>God Whispers, Stories of the Soul, Lessons of the Heart</u>.[31] In the chapter on self forgiveness, she imparts the wisdom of letting go of regrets, of the 'should have' and 'could haves,' by sharing insights gleaned from the Hebrew language. "That's what 'repentance' means in Hebrew. The word for repentance is teshuvah and it means to turn toward the right path, the path that leads to an understanding of God." The Lord is waiting with open arms to receive you in love, and "make straight" your path.

Exploration: Complete the review of last week's journal, then plan this week to reorient to True North.

1. What paths are you traveling that may become unwanted detours?

2. What did your weekly review reveal to you about yourself and your habits?

3. Is there something you experienced or accomplished that amazed you?

4. What orientations or goals will you prioritize for the coming week?

> *Fanaticism consists of redoubling your effort*
> *when you have forgotten your aim.*
> *– George Santayana*

Turning Point 4 — God's Leading

God is far more interested in your having an experience
with Him, than He is interested in getting a job done.
— Henry Blackaby

Objective: Your life is abundant and adventurous when you anticipate God's activity in and around you, and you decide to join in.

Position: God is living and active, always creating. Using the tools and information in this guide to make Higher Choices lets you fulfill your part of the co-creative process. However, knowing the Lord and doing His will are never reduced to following a formula. Your Course represents your understanding of what you can do today to begin, or continue, the adventure toward your Destination. It is your travel guide, highlighting your position on the map and the planned route. It shows scheduled pit stops, site-seeing venues, and arrival time estimates. Your plan is based upon the vision that has been revealed to you so far, which is only a portion of the larger picture. Thus, designing a life plan, certainly one designed to leave you open and receptive to the Connection and Direction God will foster, mandates flexibility. The logo on my business cards and website is my friend Wendy's interpretation of this phenomenon — two curved lines with arrows pointing up, twisted around each other. I love it! Following God's leading will never be a straight path. Your ability to go with the flow and enjoy the twists and turns will determine your success and happiness. Rabbi Karyn Kedar writes, "The twists and turns of our lives are meant to be. They teach us great truths if we can see them as part of a story that instructs.[30]"

Henry Blackaby's Bible study <u>Experiencing God : Knowing and Doing the Will of God</u>[5] teaches a sequence of seven principles that help us know God's will. Number 3 is, "God invites you to become involved with Him and His work." I learned through this study that God always takes the initiative, and I must be open and actively looking to see where God is moving. I must allow Him to develop my character. I must let Him reveal His thoughts to me. Thus, my Course will bend as I grow and follow God. It is always God's plan; He is in the lead.

We all are God's instruments. Isaiah 64:8 says, *"But now, O Lord, You are our Father; We are the clay, and You our potter."* When you truly seek to do God's will, you will be like the clay, allowing God to shape you into the vessel He requires at any particular time and place. Blackaby shows how wonderfully freeing this knowledge of God's sovereignty is, because when we come to God desiring to know what He is doing around us, we also receive the assurance that it is certain to come to pass.

The true objective of living on purpose is to connect with the people God intends for us to serve, and be served by. Connection provides new direction for our lives. Most of the time, the new direction will be an awesome opportunity we would not perceive of on our own. Jesus said, "Follow me." Go with Him, for His ways are not our ways. You may be traveling your Course quite well, requiring no 're-orientation' at all. However, do not get so caught up in reaching your Destination that you miss the beauty, excitement, possibility, or badly needed rest God offers!

Following God's lead means that you allow Him to be ahead of you, while keeping Him always within sight. Focusing on the present makes it easier to see God in your daily events and encounters.

Being receptive and responsive to the promptings of the Holy Spirit is a function of awareness. So much of our troubles come from letting our minds dwell on the past, or wonder into the future. Dale Carnegie advises his readers to "live in day-tight compartments.[10]" The moments you are spending reading this book are the only ones you have. Living is done in the present. When our minds are focused on something that happened in the past, or contemplating what might occur tomorrow, we totally miss out on true abundant life. There is a poem entitled "I Am" that states it best (as best I can remember it):

> I was remembering the past and feeling sad about regrets,
> and God said,
> "When you live in the past, it is hard, I am not there. I Am."
> I was thinking about tomorrow and feeling
> anxious about the unknown, and God said,
> "When you live in the future, it is
> hard. I am not there. I Am."

When you recognize new opportunities, remember to A.S.K., and God will make His desires known. Take time to consider what God may be leading you to do. When I was invited to participate in the prayer group mentioned earlier, I had never felt a particular calling toward intercessory prayer. My first reaction was to think that would not suit me. Thankfully, I sensed both an opportunity to learn more about prayer and serve others, particularly my friends and family, by openly sharing joys and concerns with fellow believers. Many answered prayers attest to the fruit of our labor. In addition, along with giving my time to serve others through prayer, I received great blessings from the deep bonds developed with these women. In hindsight I see that God lead me to this group, so they would be a source of comfort, encouragement, and wise counsel when I was dealing with family issues. God the Father leads His children into green pastures, beside the still waters. Do not hesitate to follow God's leading.

Exploration: Look for new or unusual insights and circumstances to see how God is at work around you.

1. God speaks to us through the scripture, the church, and our circumstance. What are you hearing?

2. Is there someone you encountered this week to whom you feel called to make a connection?

3. There are many ways to accomplish a goal. How might a new opportunity, previously not considered, be a new and exciting avenue for you that is consistent with your purpose?

> *If the Lord delights in a man's way, he makes his*
> *steps firm; though he stumble, he will not fall,*
> *for the Lord upholds him with his hand.*
> *— Psalm 37:23-24*

AUTHENTICITY

When you are content to be simply yourself and don't
compare or compete, everybody will respect you.
— Lao Tzu

Orientation 11 - God is uniquely
revealed to others through you.

Higher Choices emphasizes God's will for *you*, not others. Co-creating your life with God through the Ask, Seek, Knock process matures your relationship with God, such that you trust God to guide your daily decisions. You are free from second-guessing, able to move forward confident you are doing the right thing. You read in the Priority Orientation that regret is an emotion you feel when you act contrary to your personal values. Authentic people experience less regret and greater peace of mind, because their consistency of thought, word, and deed reflect their values. "What a rare opportunity it is to be aware of who you really are without the distractions of what others need you to be," says Karyn Kedar.

Making choices that support your purpose requires you to know yourself and be comfortable in your own skin. Each believer possesses qualities that uniquely contribute to God's greater will. Each person contributes to the world what no other can. That is what makes people so interesting. How boring it would be if we were all alike! Your uniqueness is a product of many influences, including your genes, life experiences, values, and beliefs. Yet, embracing and sharing this uniqueness is challenging.

The four Turning Points you will consider in this orientation are:

1. Creativity – Embrace your originality as the spark for creative living.

2. Courage – Move beyond your fears by taking courage from who you are in Christ.

3. Influence – Higher Choices increase your circle of positive influence, and protect you from negative influence.

4. Service – Traveling your course positions you to serve in uniquely special ways.

You will learn why being authentic is important, and how to experience its rewards. You will also understand why it can be a challenge. The easier path is to do what you see others are doing. However, your God-capacity expands every time you act in authentic love. Role models, teachers, and parents are a vital part of anyone's journey. Learn what you can from them, and then carve your own path. We must all ultimately make our own way. Dare to be authentic.

Turning Point 1 – Creativity

*I learned from her and others like her that a first-rate soup
is more creative than a second-rate painting, and that,
generally, cooking or parenthood or making a home could be
creative while poetry need not be; it could be uncreative.*
– Abraham H. Maslow

Objective: Embrace your originality as the spark for creative living.

Position: Everyone is creative - no exceptions. The words "creativity"
and "originality" are synonyms. Creativity results from originality
of thought or expression. Wikipedia states, "Although popularly
associated with art and literature, it is also an essential part of
innovation and invention and is important in professions such as
business, economics, architecture, industrial design, graphic design,
advertising, mathematics, music, science and engineering, and
teaching." The key to creativity is a willingness to be original.

God is *The Creator*. So, does it not make sense that one of the ways
you are most godlike is your wholesome creative expression, whatever
form that may take? Creativity inspires through a multitude of forms
and expressions. Many people recognize God's grandeur and majesty
in nature. The creative aspect of God is what helps me see that God
is alive and active in our world today. I see God in the positive,
inspiring, and fresh ideas of others, from the technological genius
of a medical procedure, to a beautiful piano concerto. Think about
some of your favorite things. Isn't their originality the thing that
attracts?

179

Let me tell you about my friend Wendy DiNicola. She created the Higher Choices Compass cover art. Wendy knows her mission, "to communicate and inspire creative ideas through fine art, and other art forms, in a stimulating and nurturing environment." Her art presents an astonishingly unique perspective of familiar objects and scenes. Wendy's work reveals her humor, wit, and sense of beauty. It not only shows me something about the world I otherwise would not see, it inspires me to be creative also. Of course, I simply enjoy being able to look at it every day! Although Wendy is an artist, she is also creative in parenting, working with children, decorating her home, and running a business. She is authentic in all endeavors.

Peter McWilliams said, "One of the great joys of life is creativity. Information goes in, gets shuffled about, and comes out in new and interesting ways." Find your joy by allowing your originality to guide your choices. Whether it is your approach to problem-solving, home decorating, or organizing the church music library, your original flair brings something to the world that was not there before. Let others benefit by seeing the world through your eyes.

Perhaps you have read or heard stories about one of many famous music composers or artists who reported feelings of such high creative inspiration that they felt as if there were merely an instrument of God, letting God express Himself through them. Julia Cameron calls this "channeling.[8]" "When writing is perceived as channeling spiritual information rather than inventing intellectual information, writing becomes a more fluid process that we are no longer charged with self-consciously guarding. Instead, we are charged with being available to it. We can 'plug in' to the flow of writing rather than thinking of it as a stream of energy we must generate from within ourself." Although Julia's work is directed toward writers and the joy of writing, she vehemently promotes creativity as a natural characteristic of every individual, released by all vocations and manner of human activity. She understands that the creative process is at its highest capacity, flowing most freely, when we put the ego aside.

The first time I attended a women's retreat was in the late 1980s, in Blackstone, Virginia. I have often remembered the keynote speaker's description of how she greets herself each morning by looking into the bathroom mirror over her sink, and saying to herself out load, "Good morning earthen vessel." She starts her day with a reminder to be available for God in humble receptiveness. She adopted the view St. Paul took of his ministry, that it was Christ working through him. *"For God, who said, 'Let light shine out of darkness,' made his light shine in our hearts to give us the light of the knowledge of the glory of God in the face of Christ. But we have this treasure in jars of clay to show that this all-surpassing power is from God and not from us"* (I Corinthian's 4:6-7). God created you to be an original vessel.

Exploration: Express authentic creativity in as many ways as you can.

1. List at least one way you express your originality in each of the following: home, work, leisure, and community.

2. Name 3 creative people you admire. List the specific unique attributes that contribute to their appeal.

3. What simple, original 'work' can you create today?

4. Being creative does not necessarily mean you produce something. Your style and approach in any endeavor is an original contribution. What is unique and creative about your style in parenting, socializing, serving, cooking, etc.?

The creative is the place where no one else has ever been. You have to leave the city of your comfort and go into the wilderness of your intuition. What you'll discover will be wonderful. What you'll discover is yourself.
– Alan Alda

Turning Point 2 – Courage

This soul, or life within us, by no means agrees with the life outside us. If one has the courage to ask her what she thinks, she is always saying the very opposite to what other people say.
– Virginia Wolf

Objective: Move beyond your fears by taking courage from who you are in Christ.

Position: What stifles authenticity? Fear and doubt are largely to blame. Fear of failure perhaps, or doubting your abilities. Fear of what other people may think, and doubt that anything you have to offer is of value. Authentic people exert courage to overcome these two crippling mindsets. Courage is a virtue. In the Catholic tradition, courage is one of the cardinal virtues[47], equated to forbearance, endurance, and ability to confront fear and uncertainty, or intimidation. It takes courage to remain true to your values when the world is telling you that they are outdated, or unrealistic. It takes courage to follow your dreams when uncertainty lurks and obstacles arise.

My maternal grandmother was a courageous woman. When my mother and her brother were six and five years old, their father died of jawbone cancer. In a time when working women were definitely the minority, she worked to put herself through college in order to earn a living as a school teacher. Being a single mother while having to study and work several miles away from her children presented her with many challenges: separation from her children, relying on help from her parents and other family members, managing a tight budget, and the like. She never remarried, partially because she wanted to raise her children according to her values. She had the courage to move forward and do what she thought was best despite uncertainties. Although I never had a conversation with her about her faith, I know that she was a godly woman. She put her trust in the Lord, and I am thankful for her example.

Courage is not the opposite of fear, rather the strength and determination to proceed in your Higher Choices despite that feeling. Courageous people are successful people, because they refuse to be immobilized by fear. Here is the main question you have the ask yourself: "Am I going to let fear keep me from being obedient to God, and following my dreams, or am I going to let this feeling control me?" Joyce Meyer advises her audience to be afraid and do 'it' anyway.

The word 'fear' is often described as an acronym, FEAR - False Evidence Appearing Real. You learned about the link between thoughts, emotions, and actions in the Fitness Orientation. Acknowledging that fear is simply an emotion, we can trace its origin to the thoughts we allow. You cannot eliminate fear any more than you can eliminate other emotions, however, once you identify the feeling, you can examine your thoughts to see what is feeding it. Negative and positive emotions alike must be continuously fed by your thoughts to persist. God knows this about us, of course, which is why there are so many Bible verses reminding us to "fear not."

The book of Romans is Paul's most important discourse on the subject of righteousness. Paul explains that Christ's death and resurrection demonstrates the magnitude and power of God's wondrous love. Verse 31 says, *"If God is for us, who can be against us? He who did not spare his own Son, but gave him up for us all - how will he not also, along with him, graciously give us all things?"* In addition, verses 15 and 16 state, *" for you did not receive a spirit that makes you a slave to fear, but you received the Spirit of sonship. The Spirit himself testifies with our spirit that we are God's children."* Those who believe in Jesus Christ receive God's acceptance through faith, which enables them to live boldly as heirs to the Kingdom.

Perfect love overcomes fear. 1 John 4:18 tells us, *"There is no fear in love [dread does not exist], but full-grown (complete, perfect) love turns fear out of doors and expels every trace of terror! For fear brings with it the thought of punishment, and [so] he who is afraid has not reached the full maturity of love [is not yet grown into love's complete perfection]."*

Like my grandmother, I now am beginning a new chapter of my life as a single woman and mother. I face many uncertainties and challenges. God's promises to always be with me and to care for me bring me much comfort and peace of mind. I choose to exercise faith, believe in God, and take action in line with the guidance I feel He is giving me. One scene from the movie Indian Jones and the Last Crusade[32], is a very inspiring reminder for me to act in faith. In his quest to possess the Holy Grail, Harrison Ford reaches the edge of a cliff over a cavern a mile deep. The Holy Grail is just on the other side, and he cannot believe he has come this far to fail. Despite the fact that there is no bridge or safety net, he puts all of his weight forward, stepping out into what appears to be nothingness. In the last instant, the bridge becomes visible, and he easily passes from what would otherwise be a dead end onto the path to great treasure. The treasure had been well guarded, for the fearful relinquish their prize.

I remember another movie that gave me an idea for identifying fearful, self-defeating thoughts. Originally a stage production, Neil Simon's Chapter Two features James Caan as George, a middle-aged widower struggling to escape the memory of his deceased wife. George is introduced to a soap opera star, played by Marsha Mason. In comedic Neil Simon style, romance ensues and they marry. After five years, however, George breaks off the relationship that seems to be just what he needs to enjoy life again. He does not really understand why he wants to run away from the relationship, until he recalls what his psychiatrist used to tell him. The doctor told George that whenever he felt stuck to ask himself, "What is it you are afraid will happen if …?" So, George asks himself this question. "What is it I am most afraid if…I stay with my wonderful wife?" The answer comes: "I am afraid I'll be happy." It is then, of course, that George realizes he really has nothing to fear. He may lose his second wife also, but he will enjoy many happy times with her now! That question made a lasting impression upon me. I have often asked myself that question to get unstuck. Fear is immobilizing, causing us all to get stuck from time to time. The possibility of success can often be just as frightening as the possibility of failure. Perhaps I was learning the 'power of the question' even then.

Exploration: Consider what fears and doubts may be keeping you from realizing your vision.

1. Review your goals list and assess whether your progress in one or two may be due to a lack of courage. Take one small, bold step toward that goal today.

2. List three goals in your course you have procrastinated. Give them a due date, and take the next step.

3. What original idea(s) are you waiting for permission to act upon? Whose approval do you seek and why?

4. FEAR: *False Evidence Appearing Real*. What is false about some of the fears you have?

5. How can receiving God's grace and acceptance bolster you to take bold steps to stay on Course?

One could say that the courage to be is the courage to accept oneself as accepted in spite of being unacceptable.
– Paul Tillich

Turning Point 3 – Influence

It takes tremendous discipline to control the influence,
the power you have over other people's lives.
– Clint Eastwood

Objective: Higher Choices increase your circle of positive influence, and protect you from negative influences.

Position: Everyone has the power to influence. The definition of influence is "the capacity or power of persons or things to be a compelling force on or produce effects on the actions, behavior, opinions, etc., of others." Notice that the definition uses the word "power." We all have capacity to effect what others think, say, and do by whatever we think, say, and do, for both good and bad. Consistently making Higher, authentic Choices to be consistent with God's will for you increases your God-capacity, and thus your sphere of influence. God works through people in ways we do not fully understand. He enlarges your commitment to your calling by placing you in locations and situations that serve particular people at particular times.

Connection and Direction operates through influence. Bonds between individuals naturally result in some change in both persons – they have influence over one another. As one person connects with another, each is exposed to opportunity to alter their Course and take a new direction. New direction is merely an opportunity, for each will have to choose whether or not to adopt the opinion, actions, and behaviors they encounter. I know there is something about quantum physics and energy potential to interject here, but that is way over my head!

To be authentic also means to be supported by unquestionable evidence, and entitled to acceptance or belief due to known facts, to be trustworthy. Think of a precious work of art certified as genuine, or an official report from a government agency. As you live and serve authentically, people will recognize your true talents and character, and you too will be trusted and accepted. Those who seek God with all of their heart and listen to the Spirit of Truth will be a wonderfully positive influence in this world. Second Corinthians 3:3 says, *"You show that you are a letter from Christ, the result of our ministry, written not with ink but with the Spirit of the living God, not on tablets of stone but on tablets of human hearts."* Higher Choices are positive influences.

How does being authentic protect you from negative influences? The greater the number of Higher Choices made, the fewer the number of bad choices. Staying aligned to True North is a tactic for protection from all kinds of harm. Psalm 37:23 tells us, *"If the Lord delights in a man's way, he makes his steps firm; though he stumble, he will not fall, for the Lord upholds him with his hand."* Peer pressure can be overwhelming, especially for impressionable young adults. Those who are comfortable in their own skin find it easier to say 'No' to bad influences. When you and I focus on being true to God and ourselves, we are less vulnerable to powers that distract and dissuade.

Let your light shine. Be salt. Disciples of Jesus Christ are called to be intentional about spreading the Good News, and increasing God's kingdom in the hearts and minds of their fellow man. The greater your God-capacity, the brighter and stronger your light shines. Embracing your gifts and talents and looking for every opportunity to exploit them is not egotistical. It is in fact humbling to realize, as Clint Eastwood said, that you have been given power to direct someone else's life. The paths others take are their choices, yet, your influence will affect those choices. Children are especially vulnerable to our influence. If you are a parent or teacher, or serve children in another way, your power extends beyond influence to control, simply due to your position of authority. Obviously, we must be careful with these precious little ones. If I were to ask you to name one or two persons who greatly influenced you, chances are good you would recall a teacher, coach, or other adult who cared for you, taught you a life lesson or two, and encouraged you to be your best.

One thing I love about coaching is seeing the excitement and enthusiasm my clients radiate when they discover their mission. Leading them through self-discovery by shining a little light on the possibilities of purposeful living, I am blessed to see the influence that triggers a positive change in them and their life's direction. Even greater is the way they influence me. I am enriched by their perspective on God and the world, and inspired by their passion for ministry, growth, and service.

Exploration: Be mindful of the influence you exert on those around you.

1. What habits and behaviors do you have that set a good example for others?

2. How are you influencing friends, family members, and co-workers to whom you are connected?

3. How are you allowing them to be a compelling force on you?

> *You can never really live anyone else's life, not even your child's. The influence you exert is through your own life, and what you've become yourself.*
> – Eleanor Roosevelt

Turning Point 4 — Service

How can I be useful, of what service can I be?
There is something inside me, what can it be?
— Vincent Van Gogh

Objective: Traveling your course positions you to serve in uniquely special ways.

Position: I believe there are two realms of service. One is an individual journey, where you are serving simply by living on "purpose." As you authentically offer your spiritual gifts, talents, and skills in line with your purpose, your service to others is automatic, unforced. Your personal mission and vision statements encompass your whole life, thus the people around you benefit from the activities you do at home, at work, at school, at church, and in the community. The second path is the realm of community service. It is important to be involved in group efforts. Believers are called to use their spiritual gifts in conjunction with others, because we are all members of the body of Christ. The Network[7] program mentioned in the Spiritual Gifts Turning Point states two purposes of spiritual gifts:

- Glorify God

- Edify others

Getting involved translates to meaningfulness, because you know you are contributing to others. It allows you to participate in something larger than yourself. Synergy and collaboration produce more, with greater efficiency and effectiveness. Paul's first letter to the church in Corinth describes the importance of knowing and using spiritual gifts, emphasizing God's plan that members of the church act as one body with many parts. Chapter 12, verses 12-31, illuminate the church's need for every member to contribute, because everyone performs a special function. *"The eye cannot say to the hand, 'I don't need you!' And the head cannot say to the feet, 'I don't need you!' On the contrary, those parts of the body that seem to be weaker are indispensable."* (1Cor 12:21-22). Like trying to perform "Stars and Stripes Forever" without a piccolo, one missing instrument makes the work incomplete.

Serving alongside others, whether through church, community, business, or government, is where you will experience the greatest degree of Connection and Direction. The challenge for you and I is to remain authentic to our individual calls by choosing opportunities to contribute that are in line with our respective missions. Undeniably, there are urgent needs that require the participation of every warm body and willing soul. At these times it is appropriate to step outside yourself, forsaking the 'it's not my job' attitude and the 'I don't think I'm capable' excuse to say 'yes' and get involved. However, these times are temporary. Your God-capacity is at its greatest when you stay on mission. If you are a talented theater director, then step up and direct the contemporary service drama. Resist the temptation to take on the role of lighting technician, stage designer, or whatever else another person on the team could do. Not only are you free from stress and excessive time commitments to excel at leading the cast to the most inspiring production, but you will open up opportunities for others to contribute and grow in the areas where they are gifted. Holding back out of false modesty is exactly that – false.

Spending too much time serving in the wrong capacity is a sure way to experience burnout. When my children were toddlers, we were extremely blessed to have our children nurtured and educated at our church's childcare center. Because it was part of outreach ministry, church members were asked to serve on the childcare board. This administrative body was composed of childcare professionals, church members, and parents. Being both a church member and a parent, the committee asked me to serve on the personnel committee. I served one year of my three-year commitment before deciding that that position was not a good fit for me or the board. It takes a person with gifts of mercy, encouragement, shepherding, and the like to work through work-place personnel issues with grace. I was able to contribute toward the committee goals while serving, but I experienced frustration and failure, trying to walk a path carved for someone else. Someone with the gifts listed above would contribute more. That experience is a good example of the A.S.K. process at work. Back then I did not pray about the opportunity to directly *ask* God what I should do. Still, trusting the guidance of the church's nominating committee, and wanting to help my children anyway I could, my initial *idea* was to say 'yes.' I tried out that idea, gave it some practice and persevered through 12 monthly meetings (not all bad – there were many happy, rewarding experiences). Yet, I discovered through this experience what my *truth* was, by discovering what it was not.

Life experience also plays an important role in offering authentic service. The trials and temptations you have gone through provide insight and practical wisdom to benefit others. When you are vulnerable and open enough to tell your story, you offer belonging, understanding, and hope. Others feel a sense of *belonging* simply by realizing they are not alone in their experience. You show them that not only does everyone struggle from time to time, but that you are intimately familiar with their particular struggle. You speak the same language, and thus intimate dialogue can begin; a connection forms. Giving your time and attention to serve a fellow sojourner by listening and sharing experiences lets them feel *understood*. Their feelings are validated, allowed to be released. You help them move away from what may be negative, destructive emotions to positive, restorative emotions. You give them *hope*, because you are an example of someone who made it through a similar ordeal, who overcame, who survived, now all the more stronger and wiser.

Exploration: Be intentional about seeking opportunities to serve and making them part of your Course.

1. Review your Course and estimate the percent of time you have scheduled for either individual or group service.

2. Select one person in a leadership role at your church, or in your community, to whom you can share your desire to serve and volunteer.

3. Have you identified your passion? What specific group can you begin to work with in the near future that is a natural fit with your vision (youth, homeless, battered spouses, singles, etc.)?

4. How might your personality and personal style make your gifts and talents unique?

We cannot live for ourselves alone. Our lives are connected by a thousand invisible threads, and along these sympathetic fibers, our actions run as causes and return to us as results.
– Herman Melville

RELATIONSHIPS

People who need people are the luckiest people in the world.
— Robert Merrill and Jule Styne

Orientation 12 - It's all about relationships!
The primary benefit of making Higher Choices is experiencing abundant life through your relationships. Your relationship with the living God comes first. The quality of that relationship dictates your relationship with people. In fact, I was once told that the Ten Commandments can be divided into two sections: the first four direct our relationship with God, and the remaining six direct our relationship with all of humanity. The blessings you receive from your connection with God enable you to be a blessing to others.

God made us to be relational people. We need family and friends. Creativity, service, goals, mission – what does it all matter if there is no one to share it with? You have been learning how to experience abundant life by discovering your Destination and being intentional about the adventure that will take you there. You can rest assured that your path will lead you to some miraculous, enjoyable connections. God will bring people into your life, the very people you need at the time. Likewise, you will touch someone and change their life for the better, even if only for a brief while.

The movie <u>Family Man</u>[4], starring Nicholas Cage and Tea Leoni, is a cute tale of a wealthy New York businessman who sees what his life would be like had he chosen a love relationship over the career success he now enjoys. His real life is that of a high-powered New York City executive; rich, handsome, and enjoying all that worldly success can buy. His imagined life, sort of the way Scrooge has an imagined life, is that of a happily married New Jersey tire salesman – not much money, but many rewarding relationships. His first reaction is to try to get back to his former life somehow. But in the end, it is the ordinary, middle class, suburban life he wishes he had. The fine Italian suits, fast cars, and business conquests have left him lonely.

The four Turning Points you will consider in this orientation are:

1. Communication - Maintain clear, honest, and open communication channels to sustain quality relationships.

2. Faithfulness - Honor commitments to build a solid foundation for lasting relationships.

3. Forgiveness - Mend and revitalize frazzled and broken relationships through the power of forgiveness.

4. Love - Love is always your Higher Choice.

Relationships are work. Many factors determine the quality of our relationship, however making these four a priority will make you a person others want to have in their lives. Enrich your life by enriching your relationships. You will never regret it.

TURNING POINT 1 – COMMUNICATION

The more talk, the less truth; the wise measure their words.
Careful words make for a careful life;
careless talk may ruin everything.
– Proverbs 10:19, 13:3 Message

Objective: Maintain clear, honest, and open communication channels to sustain quality relationships.

Position: Communication errors cause the vast majority of relationship problems, because they create misunderstanding. People usually act out of good intentions, or reasons that make sense to them. We speak and write what makes sense to us, often failing to take time to consider how others will interpret our words. When communication is lacking, we make assumptions and jump to conclusions to fill in the void. I know, because I tend to do this! Assumptions give birth to imaginative, erroneous thinking, which leads to hurt feelings.

You have probably heard the saying that God gave us two ears and one mouth so we would listen twice as much as we speak. The mouth and ears are our predominate communication tools. I have certainly been guilty of speaking more than I should, sooner than I should. I have failed to listen twice as much as I talk. I recall an argument I had with my husband that was a classic case of miscommunication. Great separation of both time and space (halfway across the globe and 13-hour time difference) contributed to communication issues. I learned then that relying on email is more dangerous than I had previously thought! In this particular situation, days went by without either of us making any progress on a task each thought the other was handling. Our resulting argument came during a phone conversation during which we both discovered the errors, and each self-righteously claimed it was the other's fault. The communication was too infrequent and too short, with little opportunity to connect and clarify. Assumptions were made, and feelings were hurt.

Email is a wonderful tool. Most of us do not know how to get along without it. I find email messages are only effective when composed with carefully chosen words. It should not become a regular substitute for a phone call or face-to-face chat. Yet, this is a reality of the world we now live in. Social media, text messages, and all other communication innovations have actually brought the world closer together. They enable us to be a truly global community, to reach out and establish connections never before possible. But, we must all be intentional about nurturing the important relationships with the important people in our lives with a live voice on the phone, and spending time together. Good communication involves eye contact, body language, and a personal touch.

How much pain and remorse have you endured at the hands of poor communication? When have you found that your troubles vanished as soon as you cleared up a misunderstanding? Good communication is truly a matter of working to listen more than we speak. As you and I are able to be empathetic and give people credit for good intentions, then we open our hearts enable us to open our ears. Nurture your relationships at home, work, and elsewhere by giving ample time and attention to good communication. Listen before you speak, and thoroughly read written messages. The Prayer of Saint Frances says, "O Divine Master, grant that I may not seek ... to be understood, as to understand." Yes, Lord, make it so!

Exploration: Practice putting others first in your communication with open heart and ears.

1. Call one friend this week to whom you have not spoken in several weeks.

2. Send a card or letter via "snail mail" to a family member you know could really use an encouraging word.

3. Are you spending enough time to communicate effectively with your immediate family and closest friends?

4. How many email and/or text messages do send daily? Are you reading with care, and being thoughtful in your replies?

5. What do your tone of voice and body posture communicate?

Any problem, big or small, within a family, always seems to start with bad communication. Someone isn't listening.
— Emma Thompson

Turning Point 2 – Faithfulness

I meant what I said, and I said what I meant.
An elephant's faithful one-hundred percent.
– Horton, Horton Hatches the Egg

Objective: Honor commitments to build a solid foundation for lasting relationships.

Position: Ask anyone what are the vital ingredients for lasting, quality relationships, and faithfulness would be near the top of the list. You might hear other words for it, like loyalty, commitment, and dedication for example. A review of the definitions of each of these synonyms, however, convinced me that faithfulness is the best word for Higher Choices. God is faithful. The stories of God's faithfulness throughout the Bible demonstrate how key this quality is to creating beneficial relationships. Although you may be thinking primarily of marriage, faithfulness is equally important to all other connections. Certainly, any disciple desiring to grow into Christ's likeness must demonstrate faithfulness.

How fortunate we are to have the work of Theodor Seuss Geisel, otherwise known as Dr. Seuss. This famous author of the classic children's stories <u>The Cat in the Hat</u> and <u>Green Eggs and Ham</u> always wrote his stories with a moral in mind. One of my favorite Dr. Seuss characters is Horton the elephant. Faithfulness is Horton's strong suit. In <u>Horton Hatches the Egg</u>[50], Horton perseveres despite cold winters and the ridicule of friends to remain loyal to his promise to sit on the egg. Mayzie, the lazy bird, broke her promise to return after a short vacation. Thus, it is fitting that in the end, the "elephant bird" that hatched continues a relationship with Horton, rather than its mother.

Perhaps before we can know that God is love, we must first know that God is faithful. The NIV Study Bible Concordance lists 158 verses referencing faithfulness. Some are about God's faithfulness, and some describe the faithfulness of the people, or lack thereof. This personal quality is clearly a vital ingredient for our relationship with God and one another. God is a God of promise. He honors and abides by the covenants he establishes. God shows us how to be faithful.

Every type of relationship needs faithfulness. Marriages require commitment and fidelity. Working relationships require reliability and trust. Family relationships require steady affection and kept promises. It is risky to enter into relationships. You may have been hurt by putting your trust in others, and they betrayed that trust. You may have broken promises as well. Betrayal is one of the worst emotions to experience, because it is a form of rejection. Once a trust has been broken, it takes a lot of effort to mend. Forgiveness must be given quickly; trust must be earned.

I believe authenticity is a good indicator of faithfulness. When your choices are consistent with your values, and you are not afraid to show it, others will know what to expect. Your relationships will be built upon truth. Sometimes we commit to do something that is not in line with your priorities. This becomes a temptation to break promises, because we know we will regret every minute sacrificed to it. Committing to a task you should not because you are afraid of what another will think if you said 'no,' is the same.

Today's culture promotes self-interest, the notion that individual needs are the supreme objective. That line of thinking is not consistent with the value faithfulness. Faithfulness demands sacrifice. Jesus taught us to put others' needs before our own. When we are obedient, faithfulness is one of our fruits. Remember God is faithful, and be likewise.

Exploration: Review your current relationships to see how an increase in your faithfulness and devotion can improve the connection.

1. Look up 'faithfulness' in a Bible concordance. Select and read ten verses.

2. Think of someone who betrayed your trust or broke a promise. Examine your heart to see if your attitude, words, or actions contributed to that in any way.

3. How high does faithfulness rank as a quality you desire in others?

4. Are you being faithful to yourself?

Be faithful in small things,
because it is in them that your strength lies.
– Mother Teresa

TURNING POINT 3 – FORGIVENESS

In prayer there is a connection between what God does
and what you do. You can't get forgiveness from God,
for instance, without also forgiving others. If you refuse
to do your part, you cut yourself off from God's part.
– Matthew 6:14-15, Message

Objective: Mend and revitalize frazzled and broken relationships through the power of forgiveness.

Position: Nothing separates people more than the pain, guilt, and remorse that result from transgressions against one another. We hurt others and we hurt ourselves, both intentionally and unexpectedly. Thanks be to God, through Jesus Christ, our sins are forgiven. We are able to forgive others, because He has forgiven us. Faith in Jesus' death and resurrection puts us in right standing with God, thereby restoring our relationship with the Father. Our attitude should be, "freely, freely you have received; freely, freely give.[51]" The stories of King David and the apostle Peter tell me how forgiving God is. David gave in to lust with Bathsheba, and then compounded his transgression with one bad choice after another. He committed adultery, and then lied and murdered to cover it up. Yet we know that he prospered, was highly revered, and loved by God as a *"man after God's own heart."* Psalm 51, one of the Seven Penitential Psalms, is David's humble prayer for forgiveness and cleansing after he realizes his great error. David pleads for mercy and forgiveness, after first confessing his sin. *"Have mercy on me, O God, according to your unfailing love; according to your great compassion blot out my transgressions. Wash away all my iniquity and cleanse me from my sin. For I know my transgressions, and my sin is always before me. Against you, you only, have I sinned and done what is evil in your sight, so that you are proved right when you speak and justified when you judge"* (Psalm 51:1-4). Knowing God's character to be merciful, David humbled himself and boldly asked for God's cleansing forgiveness.

Peter was the one who asked Jesus how many times we are to forgive. In Matthew 18:21-35, Peter offers an answer to his own question that he thinks in quite noble. Seven times would be a generous offering, compared to three, which was the rule at the time. Jesus' response of "seventy-seven times" (some translations state "seventy times seven") really means times without number. The verses that immediately follow recount the Parable of the Unmerciful Servant. The concluding verse says the same thing as Matthew 6:14 and John 20:23 - forgive others or you will not be forgiven. I can image that Peter thought he was magnanimous enough to carry out this command. It is ironic then, that he was the one who denied Christ three times, and in his deep remorse, found out how desperately he himself needed to be forgiven. The Good News is that he was forgiven! Neither David nor Peter was perfect, yet they are two of the most holy and honored men in our faith history. Their stories magnify God's readiness to forgive. David and Peter were both restored to their rightful relationship with God. We too are forgiven when we confess our sins with a broken and contrite heart.

It takes at least two people to form a relationship. Any time one commits a wrong against the other, forgiveness is the path to a restored relationship. Ideally, both will choose to take this route. The person who made the error must confess it, ask the other to forgive them, and forgive themselves. The person wronged must forgive and release the other person from guilt for both their sakes. If either continues to hold a grudge, there will continue to be a barrier, in the form of pain, mistrust, regret, and other emotions that prevents a total healing and renewal of the relationship. As the movie with the same title aptly describes, "It's complicated!³⁵" Blame is more easily cast than caught. Who is going to make the first move?

You cannot give what you do not have. If you have not received God's forgiveness, then you have none to give away. Both Marianne Williamson and Louis Hay touched me greatly with their individual writings concerning forgiveness. In her bestselling book, <u>A Return to Love, Reflections on the Principles of A Course in Miracles</u>⁶¹, Ms. Williamson explains how to forgive in a way that is both refreshing and practical. "Forgiveness is the key to inner peace because it is the mental technique by which our thoughts are transformed from fear to love." At first hearing, the link between fear and failing to forgive seems odd. However, as you think about it deeply, letting the Holy Spirit renew your mind, you can see that if one truly loves another with all their heart, they will see past the offense, and look with compassion upon the wounds of the offender that caused them to lash out in fear. She goes on to say, "The places in our personality where we tend to deviate from love are not our faults, but our wounds. God doesn't want to punish us, but to heal us. And that is how He wishes us to view the wounds in other people." Our egos cry out for others to pay for their wrongs, but Christ says forget about it. *"Forgive them for they know not what they are doing."* (Luke 23:34)

Exploration: Do your part in mending or improving relationships by being quick to forgive.

1. Identify one or two relationships that currently need some healing. Examine the presence of any grudge or grievance, and release it.

2. Your immediate family is your top priority. Is there a family member you need to forgive right now?

3. Have you truly received God's forgiveness? Pray for the Spirit to touch your heart and let you know you are forgiven.

4. How has focusing on forgiveness this week improved both your connections and your ability to enjoy life?

He that cannot forgive others breaks the bridge over which he must pass himself; for every man has need to be forgiven.
— Thomas Fuller

Turning Point 4 – Love

Love is like pi - natural, irrational, and very important.
– Lisa Hoffman

Objective: Love is always your Higher Choice.

Position: Love conquers all. I am pretty sure that is a line in a song; probably more than one! Love is always the right thing to do. It is not, however, always an easy task. Love is a wonderful feeling everyone needs to experience, for it is vital to life itself. Most of the time, love is a choice. It is attitude followed by action. Love is also a command. When asked, *"Of all the commandments, which is the most important,"* Jesus responded, *"The most important one," answered Jesus, "is this: 'Hear, O Israel: The Lord our God, the Lord is one. Love the Lord your God with all your heart and with all your soul and with all your mind and with all your strength.' The second is this: 'Love your neighbor as yourself.' There is no commandment greater than these"* (Mark 12:29-31).

It sounds simple, so why is it so difficult? Because, our primary focuses are not on others. We are selfish, always thinking how we can get love, or why we are not getting enough of it. Being loving is a tall order. Read again the famous passage from 1 Corinthians 13:4-7: *"Love is patient, love is kind. It does not envy, it does not boast, it is not proud. It is not rude, it is not self-seeking, it is not easily angered, it keeps no record of wrongs. Love does not delight in evil but rejoices with the truth. It always protects, always trusts, always hopes, always perseveres.*" Paul covers all the bases! There are seven things love "is," and seven things love "is not." (This kind of symmetry just gives me pause at the wonder of God's Word!)

To give is to receive. Whatever we give returns to us multiplied. I am only now discovering this truth for myself. To receive love, we must give love. Like forgiveness, love can only be given to others after you receive it for yourself. The more you seek to know God, the more you discover God's great love for you. As you receive God's love, you come to love Him in return. It was interesting for me to find that John Wesley preached the importance of faith as a means to love, making the point that faith is not an aim in of itself, but we have *faith* in order that we may have *love*. In defense of his radical preaching, Wesley writes, "What religion do I preach? The religion of love: the law of kindness brought to light by the gospel. What is this good for? To make all who receive it enjoy God and themselves: to make them like God, lovers of all, contented in their lives and crying out at their death, in calm assurance, 'O grave, where is thy victory? Thanks be unto God, who giveth me the victory, through my Lord Jesus Christ' [1 Cor 15:55,57]."[37]

Gary Chapman has written a series of books on what he calls "love languages." The first general book is entitled, The Five Love Languanges[12]. I enjoyed learning Gary's principles, because I was not aware that people need to receive love in a particular way due to personality differences. Of the five love languages – words of affirmation, receiving gifts, quality time, acts of service, and physical touch – I identified my need for quality time to feel loved. Perhaps unlike many women, I do not expect gifts as a demonstration of love. Knowing your personal love language, and that of your spouse and close relations, is important for two reasons:

1. You can effectively communicate this to your spouse and other loved ones and they will better understand how to show you love, and

2. You naturally tend to give love the way you need to receive it, thus the language of love you are "speaking" may not be understood by another. They may have a different love language.

I recommend reading one of Gary's books as a way for you to make the Higher choice of working on your love walk.

Many times we think we are loving, when in fact we really are not. Paul's description of love shows me so many ways that I have fallen short! Not every day is perfect; nevertheless, love must be given on a consistent basis for it is to be authentically and completely felt by another person.

Look at just a few of Paul's love attributes more closely:

- Love is not rude – This describes a major part of our love walk. How do I speak to others, including my body language? Have I ever said nasty words to my spouse or children during an argument? Do I have a tendency to interrupt someone while they are speaking, so I can say what's on my mind?

- Love is not self-seeking – I interpret self-seeking as putting my needs before anyone else's, consistently, in a way that is out of balance and unfair. Everything must be done my way!

- Love keeps no record of wrongs – This is really a tough one, and it ties directly to forgiveness. I cannot hold a grudge against someone, in any regard, and be loving at the same time. Total forgiveness equates to a total release of an offense, and the pain I felt because of it. Love lets it go.

- Love always protects – Obviously, we naturally protect family against attack by outside forces and common dangers. The more subtle area where I can fail to protect might be protecting others' reputations by refusing to speak ill of them behind their back, or in their presence.

- Love always hopes – To show hope for someone is to communicate that I have good expectations concerning their wellbeing and behavior. People tend to live up to the expectations that key loved ones – parents, spouses – have of them. If I routinely expect a certain person to disappoint, well, then that is most likely what I will experience - disappointment. Likewise, when I communicate hopeful expectations, I help that person grow and achieve. Hope is praise, encouragement, perhaps combined with instruction. Love as hope is the opposite of being critical.

Doing all you can to align to True North and make Higher Choices will be meaningless without love. You will have missed your Destination. God is love, thus to increase your God-capacity is to increase in love. *"If I speak with human eloquence and angelic ecstasy but don't love, I'm nothing but the creaking of a rusty gate. If I speak God's Word with power, revealing all his mysteries and making everything plain as day, and if I have faith that says to a mountain, "Jump," and it jumps, but I don't love, I'm nothing. If I give everything I own to the poor and even go to the stake to be burned as a martyr, but I don't love, I've gotten nowhere. So, no matter what I say, what I believe, and what I do, I'm bankrupt without love"* (1 Corinthians 13, 1-3, The Message).

Do all you do in love, for it is your relationships that matter most of all.

Exploration: Examine your choices to see if they are motivated by love.

1. What does it look like to love the Lord your God with all of your heart, mind and strength?

2. Whom do you find challenging to love?

3. How can loving them 'as you love yourself' improve this relationship?

> *Who would give a law to lovers?*
> *Love is unto itself a higher law.*
> — Boethius

APPENDIX

List of Values

Truth	Integrity	Honesty	Freedom
Faith	Trust	Justice	Wholeness
Honor	Obedience	Self-Worth	Integrity
Dignity	Respect	Simplicity	Peace
Positive Attitude	Self-Expression	Joy	Charity
Hope	Purpose	Grace	Discovery
Creativity	Relationships	Kindness	Service
Equality	Excellence	Nobility	Humility
Simplicity	Balance	Generosity	Giving
Vision	Competence	Reliability	Mercy
Order	Harmony	Fun	Togetherness

BIBLIOGRAPHY

1. Abraham H. Maslow. Toward a Psychology of Being, Second Edition, Van Nostrand Reinhold Company, 1968.

2. ACTS Acrostic for Prayer with Bible References, Christian Renewal Ministries, http://www.crmin.org/prayerguide/acts_acrostic.htm, October 19, 2000.

3. Allen, David. Getting Things Done, The Art of Stress-Free Productivity, Penguin Books, 2001.

4. Allen, James. As A Man Thinketh, Barnes & Noble Books, 1992.

5. Blackaby, Henry, Claude King, Experiencing God: Knowing and Doing the Will of God, Member book, LifeWay Church Resources,

6. Bonhoeffer, Dietrich. The Cost of Discipleship. Touchstone, 1959.

7. Bugbee, Bruce L., and Don Cousins. Network: The Right People, in the Right Places, for the Right Reasons, at the Right Time, Zondervan Publishing Company, 2005.

8. Cameron, Julia. The Right to Write, An Invitation and Initiation into the Writing Life, Jeremy P. Tarcher / Putnam, a member of Penguin Putnam Inc., 1998.

9. Canfield, Jack, with Janet Switzer. The Success Principles, How to Get from Where You Are to Where You Want to Be. HarperCollins, 2005.

10. Carnegie, Dale, Arthur R. Pell, and Dorothy Carnegie. How To Win Friends and Influence People, Special Anniversary Edition, Gallery Books, 1998.

11. Casting Crowns, Casting Crowns, Reunion Record, Inc., 2003.

12. Chapman, Gary. The 5 Love Languages, The Secret to Love That Lasts, Moody Publishers, 2010.

13. Covey, Stephen R. The 7 Habits of Highly Effective People, Powerful Lessons in Personal Change, Free Press, 2004.

14. Diamond, David and David Weissman. Family Man, Universal Studios, 2001.

15. Drabinsky, Garth H., and Joel B. Michaels, The Gospel of John, A Philip Saville film, Visual Bible International, Inc.

16. Dunnam, Maxie. Jesus' Claims – Our Promises, A Study of the "I Am" Sayings of Jesus, The Upper Room, 1985.

17. Dyer, Wayne W. The Power of Intension, HayHouse, Inc., 2005.

18. Dyer, Wayne W. You'll See It When You Believe It, HarperCollins, 2001.

19. Edwards, Tilden H. Jr.. Living in the Presence. Spiritual Exercises to Open Our Lives to the Awareness of God. Harper San Francisco, 1995.

20. Foster, Richard J. Celebration of Discipline, The Path to Spiritual Growth, HarperCollins, 1978.

21. Foster, Richard J. Prayer, Finding the Heart's True Home, HarperOne, and Imprint of HarperCollins, 1992.

22. Gladwell, Malcolm, Blink: The Power of Thinking Without Thinking, Back Bay Books, 2007.

23. Grant, Amy. Behind The Eyes, A&M Records, 1997.

24. Hall, Barbara (creator). Joan of Arcadia, CBS Broadcasting, Inc., 2003.

25. Hayford, Jack. Worship His Majesty

26. Hesselbein, Frances. Be * Know * Do, Adapted from the Official Army Leadership Manual: Leadership the Army Way, Jossey-Bass, a Wiley Imprint, 2004

27. Humphrey, Watts S. A Discipline for Software Engineering: 1ˢᵗ Edition, Addison-Wesley, 1995.

28. Ilg, Steve. Total Body Transformation: The Acclaimed Wholistic Fitness Personal Training System That Unites Yoga and the Gym!, Hyperion, 2005.

29. Jones, Laurie Beth. Jesus, Life Coach, Thomas Nelson Publishers, 2004.

30. Jones, Laurie Beth. The Path, Creating Your Mission Statement for Work and for Life, Hyperion Books, 1998.

31. Kedar, Karyn D. God Whispers, Stories of the Soul, Lessons of the Heart. Jewish Lights Publishing, 2000.

32. Lucas, George, and Frank Marshall. Indiana Jones and the Last Crusade, Paramount Pictures, Lucasfilms LTD, 1989.

33. Meyer, Joyce. Battlefield of the Mind, Winning the Battle in Your Mind, Warner Books, 1995.

34. Moore, Beth. Believing God Day by Day, Growing Your Faith All Year Long. B&H Publishing Group, 2004.

35. Moore, Beth. Breaking Free, Making Liberty in Christ a Reality in Life, Lifeway Press, 1999.

36. Myers, Nancy. It's Complicated, Universal Pictures, 2009.

37. Ortberg, John. The Life You've Always Wanted: Spiritual Disciplines for Ordinary People, Zondervan Publishing Company, Revised Edition, 2002.

38. Outler, Albert C.. John Wesley, (Edited by Albert C. Outler), Oxford University Press, 1964.

39. Peale, Norman Vincent. The Power of Positive Thinking. Prentice-Hall, Inc. 1978, 1952.

40. Phillips, Bill. Body-for-Life. Harper-Collins, 1999.

41. Robbins, Tony. Personal Power II, The Driving Force, audio CD set

42. Rohn, Jim. Keeping a Journal: One of the Three Treasures to Leave behind, "http://www.jimrohn.

com/index.php?main_page=page&id=1349&utm_
source=jrn-2011-01-17"

43. Retrieved from "http://en.wikipedia.org/wiki/SMART_
criteria", Categories: Project management | Acronyms |
Mnemonics

44. Retried from http://en.wikipedia.org/wiki/Johnny_
Cash, November 27, 2011.

45. Retrieved from Emotional encyclopedia topics, "http://
www.reference.com/browse/emotional+"

46. Retrieved from "http://catholicism.about.com/od/
beliefsteachings/f/FAQ_Card_Virtue.htm," January
15, 2011.

47. Rubin, Jordan S. The Maker's Diet, The 40-Day health
experience that will change your life forever, Berkley
Books, 2004.

48. Rutter, John. Requiem, Arranged by John Rutter. For
SATB Choir, Soprano Solo (Accompaniment: Organ),
Hinshaw Music Inc. 1945.

49. Sailhamer, John H. NIV Compact Bible Commentary,
Zondervan Publishing House, 1994.

50. Seuss, Dr. Horton Hatches the Egg, Random House
Children's Books, 1940.

51. Shirer, Priscilla, Beth Moore, Kay Arthur. Anointed,
Transformed, Redeemed, A Study of David, LifeWay
Church Resources, 2008.

52. Simon, Neil. Chapter Two, Sony Pictures, VHS release,
1996.

53. Stanley, Charles. The Blessings of Our Inadequacy, In Touch Early Light Devotional, Thursday October 28, 2004.

54. Tillich, Paul. The Courage To Be. Yale University Press, 1952.

55. Unknown. Freely, Freely, a Hymn.

56. Warren, Rick. 40 Days of Love Study Guide, We Were Made for Relationships, 2009.

57. Warren, Rick. A Purpose Driven Life: What On Earth Am I Here For?, Zondervan Publishing Company, 2003.

58. Wetherhead, Leslie D. The Will of God. Abington Press, 1972.

59. Wiatt, Carrie Latt, Elizabeth Miles, Portion Savvy, 30 Day Smart Plan for Eating Well, Atria Books, 1999.

60. Wilke, Richard Bryd, and Juia Kitchens Wilke. Disciple, Becoming Disciples Through Bible Study, Study Manual, Second Edition, Abington Press, 1993.

61. Williamson, Marianne. A Return to Love. Reflections on the Principles of A Course in Miracles, HarperPerennial, A Division of HarperCollinsPublishers, 1992.

62. Wonder, Stevie. Innervisions, Media Sound Studios, New York, NY; Media Sound, Inc, NY, 1973.

63. Job, Rueben. AGuide to Prayer for All God's People, The Upper Room, 1998.

CPSIA information can be obtained at www.ICGtesting.com
Printed in the USA
LVOW130116180712

290492LV00002B/2/P